The Real Life
of an Internist

OTHER BOOKS IN THE
KAPLAN VOICES: DOCTORS SERIES

The Real Life of a Pediatrician (in stores now)

The Real Life of a Surgeon (in stores Summer 2009)

The Real Life of a Psychiatrist (in stores Fall 2009)

The Real Life of an Internist

Mark D. Tyler-Lloyd, MD, MPH

EDITOR

KAPLAN) PUBLISHING

This publication is designed to provide accurate and authoritative information in regard to the subject matter covered. It is sold with the understanding that the publisher is not engaged in rendering legal, accounting, or other professional service. If legal advice or other expert assistance is required, the services of a competent professional should be sought.

While the stories in *The Real Life of an Internist* are based on real events, names, places, and other details have been changed for the sake of privacy.

Published by Kaplan Publishing, a division of Kaplan, Inc.
1 Liberty Plaza, 24th Floor
New York, NY 10006

Printed in the United States

Library of Congress Cataloging-in-Publication Data

The real life of an internist / Mark D. Tyler-Lloyd, editor.
    p. ; cm. -- (Kaplan voices)
  ISBN 978-1-4277-9964-7
 1. Internal medicine--Personnal narratives. 2. Internists--Personnal narratives. I. Tyler-Lloyd, Mark. II. Series: Kaplan voices.
  [DNLM: 1. Internal Medicine--Personal Narratives. 2. Physicians--Personal Narratives. WB 115 R288 2009]
  RC48.R385 2009
  616.0092'2--dc22

                              2009001272

10 9 8 7 6 5 4 3 2 1
ISBN-13: 978-1-4277-9964-7

Kaplan Publishing books are available at special quantity discounts to use for sales promotions, employee premiums, or educational purposes. Please email our Special Sales Department to order or for more information at *kaplanpublishing@kaplan.com*, or write to Kaplan Publishing, 1 Liberty Plaza, 24th Floor, New York, NY 10006.

DEDICATIONS

To my parents, the late Reverend Nathaniel Tyler-Lloyd and Mrs. Portia Tyler-Lloyd, whose prayers and sacrifice allowed me to fulfill my dream of becoming an internist.

And to Dr. Melissa M. Freeman, my internist, who inspired me to become a physician when I was a little boy.

CONTENTS

INTRODUCTION

Mark D. Tyler-Lloyd, MD, MPH

AN INTERNIST, PLAINLY put, is a physician who specializes in internal medicine, often referred to as "adult
medicine." Training in internal medicine provides the
skill for the diagnosis, treatment, management, and prevention of a vast spectrum of adult diseases. An extensive
fund of medical knowledge and an aptitude for problem solving are essential (but not necessarily sufficient)
requirements. In a broader context, internal medicine is
the parent of more than 15 subspecialties—each of which
demands layers of further study and training, but from
which the requisite knowledge and fulfillment of exper-
tise in internal medicine must first be established.

This book examines the life, the real life, of an internist. It illuminates the experiences of those at various stages
of a rugged and rewarding journey and offers the reader
a penetrating view into the private but unusual world of
the provider—openly and candidly described. From medical student to medical resident, to private practitioner and
subspecialist, this book is an authentic review of an existence few enter and even fewer understand. The stories
contained herein replicate the unique environments that

are characteristic of the internist's world, and remind the reader that sickness, suffering, dying, and death are both foes and companions of life—but always the rival of the internist. Whether treating patients in an exclusive, elite academic institution, a regular outpatient clinic, or even a small, austere rural hospital, providing quality patient care amid the obstacles of disease, defiance, and overwhelming difficulties truly defines the internist.

Within these essays, the variety of patient encounters are vividly portrayed through the lens of both doctor and patient, and the physician-patient relationships are eloquently and elegantly depicted—terrifying and terrific at the same time. The strength of this physician-patient relationship allows doctors to help new patients, even with medical issues that require specialized care beyond the internist's training. Likewise, this powerful relationship reflects the fusion of many tender attachments and tasks often indistinguishable from one another: healer, advisor, advocate, counselor, consultant, and confidante. It is an awesome bond that connects the two with a most precious and treasured agenda: the quality of health and life. As a result, the reader will come to appreciate the internist's responsibility as much more than a career and far greater than an occupation. For as one author claims, it is a calling: a pressing beckoning from deep within for which one is chosen. And when answered, the experience is meaningful, stressful, agonizing, and mysteriously fulfilling.

This book underscores the poignant fact that the practice of medicine has as much to do with practice as with medicine. Therefore, these honest portrayals reveal mistakes as well as miracles and illustrate the complexities of multiple diseases, the challenges of ethical dilemmas, and the powerful therapeutic effects of a touch and the simple act of listening. From these stories the reader will be reminded that the physician is, above all, human—so capable, talented, skilled, gifted, and courageous, yet so vulnerable, broken, weary, wounded, and oftentimes more fearful than fearless. The reader will witness, through the words of these dedicated practitioners, genuine frustrations, surreal panic, real doubt, humility, humiliation, triumph, tragedy, and the compelling paradox of compliant patients with complaining families or rebellious patients with supportive relatives, as well as the plight of those who have no one and struggle more with isolation than with illness.

The sincerity of the stories within this book brings to light those delicate challenges which are inescapable themes in the life of an internist. Among them, it will be revealed that the internist's life has nearly as much to do with death as with life. As caretakers of adults, internists are frequently challanged with infirmities that are chronic, ongoing, and longstanding. Many of them we do not cure but desperately try to slow: high blood pressure, diabetes, and illnesses of the heart, liver, kidney, and other vital organs. Even when the collective efforts of both doctor and patient reduce or halt ailments to a stalemate, eventually all things must surrender to time. The young and the healthy ultimately age, slow down, and inevitably succumb to end-of-life issues. It is this aspect of the internist's life and lifestyle that cause the deepest wounds and richest rewards. Inasmuch as the physician is committed to the preservation of life, the death of a patient is a constant reality. And yet, at the interface of life and mortality, our patients teach us the fortune of life and of dignity in death. And, to that end, we become better physicians and better humans.

The Real Life
of an Internist

Beyond the White-Coat Ceremony

Maya Salameh, MD

M RS. HERNANDEZ DOESN'T speak English, and Jenny is not here. Sometimes I think the entire clinic would fall apart if Jenny didn't take the bus every day to translate for the helpless doctors taking care of the large Spanish-speaking patient population. But she's not here today, and Mrs. Hernandez is waiting. I'll make do with my broken Spanish. I walk in and introduce myself. She seems pleasant enough.

This will be a quick one, I think to myself, an "in-and-out" type of visit. I start by asking her the reason for the visit. That's mistake number one. The ailments come out one after another, and before I know it, I've got a case of "total body *dolor*" (total body pain) on my hands. I can't handle it. I'm post-call; I'm tired. I can't go through with this. My mind drifts, and I watch Mrs. Hernandez speaking earnestly, pointing to her neck, her back, her stomach, her legs, wincing, frowning, moaning. She's coughing, too, she says. She's been coughing for a year. I scan her chart while she talks. Ten urgent visits in the past two years for this cough. Chest X-rays have been ordered, ACE inhibitors have been taken off and put back on, Robitussin with and without codeine has been prescribed. But this cough persists.

However, I notice she has not coughed once since she started speaking. I start to feel impatient. Before I know it, I don't believe her anymore. So when she points to her right upper quadrant, wincing in pain, and tells me she has an "inflamed liver," I feel like I've had enough.

"Mrs. Hernandez, Señora Hernandez, please sit over here, *sientese aquí*; I'd like to examine you." I can tell she's not finished talking, but I'm finished listening.

She hobbles over to the exam table, wincing in pain, clutching at her back as she limps across the room. Once she is seated, I approach her, and while pulling out my stethoscope, I notice little red marks on her chest called spider angiomatas. These are classic for patients with cirrhosis—advanced liver disease. I ask her about a history of liver problems; I had not seen a mention of it in her chart.

"I was about to tell you," she says, "I was about to tell you about my inflamed liver."

I don't know what to say. I sit her back down, take a deep breath, and pull out my pen, and the real visit begins. Now I'm listening, but I feel as though I've already failed her.

* * *

Mr. Pratts is crying. His entire 380-pound frame is shaking, and he is sobbing like a baby. His legs are swollen again, and he can't get out of the wheelchair because his knees give way. He's fighting with his lover.

"My life is out of control, doctor; I don't know what to do."

I look at my watch. I'm an hour and a half behind, and I have two patients waiting. It's going to be a long afternoon. My pager goes off—it's the inpatient ward; it must be important. I ignore it.

"Have you seen your therapist recently, Tony?"

He tells me through his tears that he stopped going there. I listen and I say nothing. The minutes go by. Sheila, the head nurse, knocks on the door.

"Doctor, Mrs. Rivera is going to leave if you don't see her now."

"Well, I can't see her now, Sheila; she'll have to wait."

Tony is still crying, but he's calming down. We talk about adjusting his medications to help with his swollen legs, and he likes the idea. We talk about increasing his insulin to better control his blood sugar level. We talk about weight loss, but Tony is beyond weight loss. And I know that at this weight, we're fighting a losing battle.

We can tweak the Lasix and the insulin and the Neurontin, but Tony will never really get better. At least that's what I think as I watch him catch his breath between sentences. But I don't tell him that, because that would break him. Tony is calm now.

"Thank you doctor," he says. "Thank you for listening."

"It's my job, Tony. That's why I'm here."

* * *

Tommy was back in jail last week. They released him yesterday morning, and his first phone call was to the clinic to make an appointment with me. I know why he's here, and I brace myself as I enter the room.

"I'm in lots of pain, doc. I need my meds."

Tommy is 45 years old, and for some reason, he made some wrong decisions in the past. He can't recall which started first: the cocaine or the heroin. The drinking came next. Now hepatitis C and alcohol have ravaged his liver. Today, he is clean of drugs but in constant pain, dependent on narcotics. We've done multiple imaging studies that have revealed no obvious cause for Tommy's persistent abdominal pain.

The story changes every time. *I need my refill early because my car was broken into and they took all my stuff, including my pills. I need another refill because I lost the script you gave me, and now I've had to double up on the pills I had at home because the pain is so bad. I just need more pills, doc.*

I start to feel frustrated again. I think back to my first day of medical school, to the white-coat ceremony I'd attended in eager anticipation of my life as a doctor. I'd walk into clinic in the morning and cheerfully greet the nurses while putting on my white coat. I'd diagnose and treat. My patients would get better, and they would feel like I'd helped them because I'd ordered the right imaging study or prescribed . . .

"Doc, are you listening?"

Tommy has been speaking for several minutes, and I find myself again caught in a quagmire of stories that have no beginning and no end. I know what Tommy wants from me. And I know I have to say no because he is addicted.

"I can't give you any more pills, but I'd like to help you, Tommy."

He is angry, and the look of desperation in his eyes strikes me. I stand my ground, but I already know he'll be back tomorrow.

* * *

Walter stands up as I walk in and extends his hand with a big grin on his face. He is a healthy man in his mid-50s whom I have been treating for three years for uncomplicated hypertension. He comes every few months; we check his blood pressure and adjust his medications, and then we spend the rest of the time talking about his job or something of interest in the news. There is no reason to think today will be any different. Walter's blood pressure is good, and I tell him to keep up the good work. As I'm preparing prescriptions for his refills, I ask whether there's anything else bothering him.

"Not really, doc. I feel pretty good except for this diarrhea I've been having."

"Tell me about the diarrhea, Walter."

"It's been going on for a couple of months, no big deal really, just having it a few times a week; in between, everything is normal."

I ask him whether he's lost weight, and he thinks he may have but doesn't have a scale at home so it's hard to tell. Now he's on the examination table, and as I examine his belly, I find myself expecting it will be normal, so I'm surprised when I press down on the left side and feel something hard. I press down again. It's still there. I pause.

"Is everything okay, doctor?"

"I'm just examining you, Walter. Don't worry, just examining."

I know at that moment that this is bad news for him, but I say nothing. The rectal exam is next, and I insert my finger; again, I encounter a hard, rocklike mass. My heart sinks.

"Well, Walter, we need a CT scan and a colonoscopy."

"But why?" he asks, and suddenly he is full of questions that I do not answer.

The next day, Walter has a CT scan of his abdomen and pelvis, and I get the page from the radiologist in the afternoon. Walter has a large mass in his colon, he says;

it looks like a neoplasm. Neoplasm. Malignancy. Cancer. That's what I thought.

"Walter, I need to see you in clinic tomorrow afternoon to talk about your test results."

I hang up the phone. He's coming tomorrow at 1:00 P.M., and for first time since Walter has been my patient, I'm dreading his visit.

* * *

Ms. Moore wants me to call her Lucy. I've never met her before; she's not one of my regular patients. I'm seeing her today because she's having pain in her feet. I examine her. Her feet, apart from being dirty, look normal to me.

"Well, we'll do some blood tests, Lucy."

"But what about the pain, doctor? I can't walk."

I tell her to take Motrin, and she responds with the familiar "I've already tried, and it doesn't work."

"What about Tylenol?"

Same answer. I don't know anymore. I have no idea what's wrong with Lucy's feet. Morning clinic is over, and the other residents are gone. I'm supposed to be at noon conference. Before I know it, Lucy is teary-eyed.

"What's wrong, Lucy?"

She gives me a glimpse into her life. Her husband left her. She has no children. No one wants to have anything to do with her, she says. She was reading the Bible and talking to God and that was helping, but yesterday, in a moment of despair, she asked God if he was still listening and he didn't answer. Even God didn't answer.

"Lucy, are you thinking of hurting yourself?"

She's clutching at the Kleenex I handed her, and her eyes are fixed on the floor. She doesn't answer.

"Lucy, we need to get you some help. I'm going to ask a psychiatrist to talk to you."

"I don't want a psychiatrist," she assures me. "I'll be fine. This has been going on a long time; it'll be all right."

I convince her that this is the right thing to do, but I already know she has no choice. I step out of the room to call the psychiatric emergency room. When I return, she is gone.

"Where did Ms. Moore go?" I ask the nurses. No one knows. We search everywhere, but she is gone. We call the police. We call her home. We are unsuccessful. This is my fault.

An hour later, the phone in triage rings, and Sheila picks up.

It's Lucy. "Please tell that young doctor I'll be all right," she says. "I won't hurt myself; I've been like this for years. That doctor, she just took me too seriously is all."

"Lucy, wait, let me get the doctor to speak to you."

I reach for the phone, but it's too late. Lucy has already hung up.

The ICU

Himali Weerahandi

LIKE MANY OTHER fourth-year medical students, I didn't look forward to my intensive care unit (ICU) rotation. I dreaded the prospect of getting up early, putting in long days, presenting in front of a large team, and getting ambushed with questions. But more than that, I dreaded being in a place where patients were hooked up to breathing machines and getting fed through tubes, unable to move or talk.

We extend life, but what kind of life is it, being tethered to a machine, moving in and out of consciousness? As a third-year student, I had already seen two people in the ICU die miserable deaths, and I hadn't even done a rotation there yet! It seemed like a place filled with despair, where patients seemed to be on the brink of death, yet not allowed to die peacefully.

My first couple of days in the ICU were tough. I saw that patient management was more complicated and the patients were much sicker than I'd anticipated. The field of critical care is a relatively new field itself, a nod to the technologies it employs. But it turned out that the ICU wasn't a completely hopeless place where brain-dead people were artificially kept alive, as I'd feared. Still, ethical dilemmas do come up frequently. Most people, when asked, would say that they would not want to be hooked up to a machine to be kept alive. After the Terri Schiavo controversy, in which family members battled for years over whether the patient would have wished to be kept alive in a persistent vegetative state, more people started thinking about living wills and health care proxies—and what they'd want to be done (or not done) in the event they were ever incapacitated.

However, if health care professionals don't know that the patient has such a document outlining Do Not Resuscitate (DNR) stipulations, our job is to resuscitate a patient in distress, by any means necessary. One patient who came to us during my ICU rotation was a 77-year-old woman with multiple health problems, including diabetes. Let's call her Ms. B. She was what some would describe as "noncompliant"—she never checked her blood sugar levels and took her insulin haphazardly. Such patients can be frustrating, but I'd venture to guess that older people are sometimes noncompliant because they expect to die in a few years and want to enjoy the remainder of their life. Also, checking blood sugar does require a pinprick to the finger as well as a needle injection of insulin, and many people simply hate needles.

Ms. B was brought in to the emergency department by her family, essentially because she was acting strangely—she was not her usual self. The Emergency Department (ED) doctors soon discovered that her blood sugar was sky high and her blood pH was very acidotic, so she needed to be admitted to the hospital right away. While she was in the ED, a code was called because she went into cardiac arrest—essentially, her heart stopped beating for 45 minutes. This should be enough to kill someone, but since she was in a hospital, the ED docs shocked her and finally got a heartbeat back, after giving her practically half the drugs in the code cart and then intubating her.

Afterward, Ms. B's family informed the medical team that the patient had a legal document outlining DNR measures, which informed the reader that in a life-threatening event, she did not want to be shocked or placed on a breathing machine. The ICU team was critical of the ED docs, angry that they didn't find this out until after the fact, especially since the patient had coded for 45 minutes and likely had very severe brain damage as a result of lack of effective blood flow to the brain for so long. But perhaps it's easy to criticize when you're on the outside looking in. Being in the moment, you don't stop and ask whether the patient wants to be saved, especially if your job is to save lives. Patients come to the hospital for a reason, and one must make assumptions in situations like this because every second counts.

When Ms. B came up to the ICU, I was on the team taking care of her. As I read over her chart, my resident turned to me and said, "So, she's brain-dead, you know. There's no way she's going to wake up, after coding for 45 minutes." Then, after a moment, he emphatically added an afterthought: "Other than an act of God!" We went through the motions to officially label her as brain-dead, and we expected to withdraw care soon. We consulted Neurology for a prognosis. The family brought in the patient's DNR papers.

There are different levels of Do Not Resuscitate status, and depending on the institution, these different levels mean different things. The levels define the types of resuscitative measures the patient would receive in the event of cardiac or respiratory arrest, what types of interventions the patient would receive, and whether or not care should be withdrawn.

Despite this written documentation of Ms. B's wishes to not be connected to a breathing machine or to receive medicine to sustain a viable blood pressure, among other things, she continued to be treated with these measures because we did not have the paper documenting these wishes in our hands at the time such decisions needed to be made. At the same time, Neurology informed our team that their protocol was to give a prognosis 72 hours after the "event"—in her case, the cardiac arrest. Her family wanted to wait to see what they said, and actually changed her code status from DNR to "full code," which would allow for aggressive efforts to sustain Ms. B's life.

One morning, before these 72 hours had expired, I went into her room to examine her. I opened her eyelids to see if her pupils reacted to light, as this would indicate some level of brain activity. When I let go of her eyelids, I noticed they didn't close all the way. I thought to myself that it almost looked as if she was awake. As I continued to examine her, I noticed she seemed somewhat responsive. I placed my fingers in her hand and asked her to squeeze them. I was floored when she actually did it. I said her name—and she responded by raising her eyebrows. She was very weak, but she wasn't brain-dead. She was waking up.

She made a slow but steady recovery. Every day she was a little more awake. She weaned off the breathing machine and started breathing on her own. She weaned off the pressors, and then she didn't need to be in the ICU anymore. She was sent up to the floors on the weekend, when I wasn't in. I was told she had started talking and was feeding herself.

Is she totally back to normal? It's impossible for me to say because I don't know what her baseline was, and frankly, I don't know what she's like now. But the fact of the matter is that despite our assumption that she was brain-dead, based on the story given to our team, she had gotten better. I guess the moral of the story is that you never know. The ICU does have a lot of terminal cases, but some people do get better. Whether the majority of patients are able to achieve a good quality of life coming out of the ICU is a matter of debate, but it is clear that all those machines that artificially extend life may also act as a bridge to allow someone to heal.

WALKING THROUGH
MICHAEL REESE

David A. Matuskey, MD

I ARRIVED JUST TEN days ago, a traveler with a purpose. As a medical student who had spent his initial years in a Caribbean school, I am now on a North American tour to find the best possible hospital for my return to medicine. This tour includes cities worthy of the back of a T-shirt: New York, Atlanta, Washington, Baltimore, St. Louis, and San Francisco, just to name the major ones. This is the first leg: internal medicine in Chicago.

Tonight, I'm in Michael Reese Hospital. Lore has it that is was once the largest hospital in the United States, complete with lakefront property and a neoclassical facade. In between north and south Chicago, it was well fed with the rich arteries of prestige and money, back in the early years. Since then, the ebb and flow of the Second City had turned it into no-man's-land, a purgatory between the haves and have-nots. Despite fate's downturns, the name still conjures memories of the days when the marble foyer sparkled. For those patients with bad luck and little else, or for medical personnel with much to prove, it's still a hospital. That's why I'm here.

I'm on call. Every fourth night, I abandon my rented confines for the deserted building of the hospital with an area made up for the young doctors and the even younger students. It's on the second floor. We don't know much about the higher floors, because the elevator won't stop there and the stairwell doors are locked. The second floor was once a cardiac care unit, its dedication and formal name still ingrained on the wall. Dark wood around the entrance and carpeted floors give an executive appearance to the floor.

The nurses' station seems like it's been deserted for decades. A peach counter supports an old rotary phone with no dial tone, empty chart racks, and one old computer that on occasion can give email or patient lab values. This floor has the same unmistakable character as the rest of the hospital: aged luxury. It reminds me of a sub-vintage Lincoln Town Car, with cracked leather, faded paint, and the damp preformed bucket seats of previous owners. A vessel that's too large for the road, yet somehow it continues to ramble.

I'm part of the team which consists of Raj the resident, Ayesha and Praia the interns, and the Harvard-educated attending physician, Dr. Smith, who's been here since the hospital's good days. It's late in the evening, though, and he's gone. The resident is the one who knows the game. He also knows the spots to sleep—he's gone for long stretches, and then calls or just shows up like an apparition. I mostly follow. Second floor, sixth floor, auxiliary building floor 5, auxiliary building floor 6, radiology, coronary catheterization laboratory, and walk, walk, walk.

Our patients are as varied as the medicine we have studied. They rotate in and out of the hospital, much like us, albeit faster, and the heart, lung, bone, and other visceral patients are shipped out—before the fourth day if possible. Patient intake takes place, the call days, and if the patients stay, they complicate our lists. Nobody wants that. The newest doctors have this problem, the kept patients, and soon they are swamped.

Despite the cold and snow, it's spring—and that means that the teams are seasoned, even if I'm not. The patients have been released by my on-call day—not by magic or divine intervention, but by practicality. Except for two.

I'm talking to one now, Jesse James. He hasn't made the cutoff because his prognosis is bleak—renal cell carcinoma, a type of cancer that affects the kidneys. This is his third on-call cycle, and he's my unofficial first patient. He hasn't revealed his name, but is quiet and cordial, with manners from a long-gone era. Even at the height of his pain, he replies with a "yes, sir" or a "thank you, doctor" to the team or to me, when I see him every day in the early glow of the sunlight. I follow him closely to make sure certain key chemicals in his bloodstream are in proper balance, write prognosis notes, and try to act more experienced than my short white coat would suggest.

It's late and I'm lying in the call room after rounds. A light is on in the bathroom so I won't sleep too heavily and miss something important. The call room is a converted patient's room, still made up of two single-width beds, with a TV with hand knobs, useless to me without a remote control. Above the bed, within arm's reach, hovers oxygen and a vacuum hookup with two other outlets of unknown importance. Beyond that lies a wood structure that curtains the long light tube inside. When on, it blocks the impersonal rays and gives an effect of softening the mood. Its switch is connected to a long string, and beside it for half the way dangles the call line. I wonder briefly if anyone is on the other end of the line. Despite the distractions of these surroundings, I lie trying to sleep with the squawk and outcry of the waterproof mattress.

The intercom goes off. *Code blue, code blue in tower 2, floor 4.*

Eyes half open, I put on my shoes and coat and run down the vacant halls and up the worn stairs. I'm on the floor when I see a swarm of activity. In the room, on the bed is Jesse James. His clothes are half off, and wires and sensors are being placed for registering his vital signs. Raj and the team arrive, and we jump to advanced cardiac life support mode. I man the chest compressions component of cardiopulmonary resuscitation; Raj is the captain, efficiently barking orders to everyone around.

"Is he breathing?"

"Quick, bag him."

"Pulse."

The heart monitor has the static drone of no activity, in contrast to the whirl of scrubs, carts, and packaged equipment being ripped open.

"He's in asystole. Load first epi."

"First epi given," the nurse says.

"Stop CPR."

"Anything?"

"Nothing," replies the nurse.

"Resume compressions."

"Let's get femoral access."

"I'll try," says the intern.

"Load second epi."

"Epi ready," one of the nurses replies.

"Hold for the third minute. Who's taking the record?"

"I am," speaks up another nurse from the side.

"Okay, tell us when it's time."

Everyone is on automatic pilot at the stations, working to save Jesse.

I am still doing the compressions, nestled in an ever-smaller space in the crowd. Both interns are semi-gowned, each working on a leg as they try to unclothe Jesse for better access. This reveals urine, feces, and blood. By now, I am sweating with the labor of the living. I notice it beading around my hairline and then slowly moving down my forehead before finally launching off my nose. The sweat mixes with all the fluids—the ones that had been so carefully measured before—disappearing into the waste upon the bed.

On the next push, I hear the cracking of ribs. I look for a grimace of pain, Nature's last resolve. Nothing.

"Three minutes since last epi," calls the nurse in the back.

"Give next epi," responds Raj.

We wait motionless, hovering over this feeble body on the precipice of death. I see the patient's eyes dilate with hazy cataracts. Does he see me now? When is the true moment of death? Are we conscious at that time? Is he conscious now?

He is the first man I have seen die. These walls have seen so much birth and death, so much sorrow and joy, a century of experience—and there I am, with nothing more to offer than my initiation.

A nurse turns off all the lights except for the one above his bed, a nonverbal clue that this is now a wake. As people solemnly leave the room, life seems to slowly drain away. I am now the last one, alone with a body in a darkened room—just Jesse James, Michael Reese, and me.

Raj sees me through the door and tells me that we have to move on—it's still early. We tend to the other patients on the floors. A few hours later, we circle back to Jesse's floor. The interns are finishing the paperwork: death certificate, progress notes, and a letter for Jesse's son excusing him from work the next day. We gather as a team again, with a list of patients to care for.

We take the elevator this time and see Jesse's son. He has pushed the up button by mistake. Raj says, "Mr. James." The son turns around, listless. Raj looks at him and, with a stumble, says, "I'm, umm, sorry, you pushed the wrong button. Well . . . actually, I'm sorry about, you know . . . well . . . forget about it." Here the senior resident, who had managed all required competencies and could recite Harrison's textbook down to the exact page and paragraph, has found his failure. He pushes the down button for Jesse's son as we go up on the next carriage.

Raj was right, about the night, that is—it is a long night, and the team does not sleep.

When light finally breaks, I am alone in one of the endless corridors with brown subway tiles and oxidized window frames. The steel radiators form their own ecosystem, insulating the hospital from the numbing blast skipping along the cold and pale "third coast" of the Great Lakes. I want that blast to finally leave these veteran doors and allow the wind to channel through the forgotten urban valleys and curl around the senses. As I walk past each window, I deliberately step into the rays of light cast onto the floor. The janitor, prompt as any doctor, is tending to his duties at the end of the corridor. He is polishing the last square of light when we meet. In my short tenure here, we have found our customs in weather talk.

"It's a windy one today," he says to me, still mopping the floor.

"Believe it or not, I'm ready for it."

"Why, Doc? Was it a tough one last night?"

"Yes."

He looks up at me with a smirk and says, "You know, you do look like the walking dead today."

"Yes," I say as I smile back. "But at least I'm still walking."

HIGHER POWER

Eliezer Van Allen, MD

D URING THE CLINICAL years of medical school, your average medical student is expected to take a lot of time getting to know patients intimately, spending long amounts of time with them in order to truly know them. On most rotations you are generally assigned only one to three patients at a time, so there is often ample time to give them the attention they, in most cases, deserve. So much of healing, they are taught, seems to revolve around the simple act of sitting down at a patient's bedside, listening to the patient's story, and performing a physical exam (although a squirt of antibiotics or a snip of an appendix can help from time to time as well).

This makes it all the more ironic that perhaps the greatest challenge in the transition from medical student to intern (or resident, or attending for that matter) is that the precious element of time is taken away, and the physician has to deal with this without compromising patient care. What started as a 30 to 60 minute encounter progressively shrinks, to the point that at peak efficiency, any self-respecting intern can probably limit actual face time encounters with a patient to less than five minutes—and still extract enough information to guide the course of therapy and interventions for the day.

I bring this up because over the course of my intern year, one factor has become alarmingly clear: namely, that an increasing number of patients are distrustful, antagonistic, doubtful, and angry with health care providers. I can rattle off a lengthy list of patient encounters that involved stacks of (often false) information patients printed out from the Internet, with the patient angrily shaking the papers in the doctor's face when the doctor does not agree with whatever crap some quack on the Internet typed up. Then there are patients that repeatedly insist on seeing only specialists and/or attendings, even though they know they are at a teaching hospital and have absolutely no choice about whether the intern or medical student sees them on rounds every day. I think a lot of these encounters can be easily fixed, but the system no longer allows us to spend the time necessary to do so, which then contributes to the declining respect for physicians in our society.

I had not thought much about this until today, because until today I really had nothing to compare this antagonistic relationship to. However, this afternoon I met a very pleasant and exceedingly tragic young man who is dying from cancer. Stoic but occasionally tearful, he ended up in our hospital after vomiting blood at the airport shortly after arriving from his home country of India on a business trip. My encounter with him was somewhat standard; it was my encounter with his mother, who hopped on the first plane to America upon hearing her son was in the intensive care unit (likely at some obscene financial cost), that was so remarkably unusual.

With an unusual amount of time on an abnormally quiet day, I was actually able to carry on a lengthy discussion of the patient's case with his mother. After I discussed the case with the patient and his mom, the mother started talking about her concerns regarding his health, repeatedly invoking the notion that God will help her son, that God will cure his cancer, that God will ease his pain. After a few minutes of this monologue, she turned to me and said, "And honestly, we both know that God is too busy to meddle in the day-to-day health of all the souls on this earth. That is why you are here . . . you are the hand of God, to do his bidding . . . you are God." She grabbed my hand and repeated, "You are God."

I smiled, held her hand for a few moments, and after a brief discourse walked outside the room to take a deep breath. I remember thinking that this had to be one of the most, if not *the* most, awkward patient encounters I experienced in my budding career, more frustrating than my experience with a drug addict who called me a "pain-medicine Nazi."

After all, I spent most of the year being reminded by patients about how idiotic I am, how incompetent the hospital staff has become, and how incomprehensible the system shall always be. And here I am, being proclaimed God so matter-of-factly, so nonchalantly—by someone who held her oncologist from India in the same regard, and does not appear to understand that neither one of us is going to be able to cure anything her unfortunate son has, before it takes his life.

At first, after walking back to the resident room, I recall thinking, "Well, it's about damn time someone appreciated what I do all day!" It was so refreshing to be put on that pedestal because, obviously, there is no other pedestal that quite matches up to the one God (or the athiest all-powerful equivalent) is on. But it was only a few moments later that I started feeling extremely uncomfortable. Would a physician prefer the current state of medicine in our society, one rife with distrust, conflict, and frustrations? Or would a physician prefer to return to the extremely paternalistic state in which the physician was king, immediately trusted, the ultimate arbiter of life and death?

At first, the answer may seem obvious to those of us operating under the current mode of existence. Frankly, I would not be shocked if, the next time a patient comes in with a stack of information printed out from some quack website, questioning a doctor's every move and shoving those pieces of paper in his or her face, the doctor may simply say, "Fine, if you want to take the Internet's advice over mine, that's okay; just don't come to see a doctor or go to a hospital ever again." (Right before the doctor takes that stack of papers and throw them down the hall.)

Fortunately, we don't have to imagine what a return to the days of strict paternalism might be like; we have the vast majority of modern medicine to guide us. After all, the Tuskegee experiment and the Nazi medical crimes were both done under the idea of the all-knowing, all-powerful physician. Yet those are admittedly extreme examples that are perhaps more a reflection of the stunning depths of humanity, of how even medicine can be twisted into something evil, and not a particular aspect of paternalistic medicine itself.

At a more practical level, it is important for me to express the intense discomfort that swept over me shortly after that patient encounter. Before I became a doctor, I went through an incredible series of silly hoops, whether they were exams, activities, or hour upon hour of incredibly obnoxious interactions with awful people. In fact, my education over the last four years does not exactly prepare me for . . . well . . . much of anything, as it turns out. And I feel very confident in saying that nothing I went through actually amounts to any true higher stature, and surely no true higher power.

Most important, I have learned that it is far better to be humiliated, scorned, and distrusted in the current medical system than to be falsely idolized in the older model. So much of this past year has been about accepting failure, whether it manifests itself in the cancer-ridden body of a previously healthy 40-year-old with a wife and two young kids, or in the glazed eyes of a crack addict with a habit I will never get him to break. In the wake of these perpetual failures, the notion that physicians are somehow elevated in society holds no ground—and I think it is silly for any physician to attempt to embrace this persona. This new self-perception is something medical students are now taught to varying degrees, but my hunch is that these lessons last as long as it takes for most newly minted doctors to find themselves in a similar position to mine: weighed down by a year's worth of sometimes literally being shit on, only to be elevated to godlike status by kind (if misguided) patients—and enjoying the latter role far more than the former. The attitude starts there and only grows.

Where to go from here? As with most things, moderation seems like the key. I think most doctors would willingly give up a fair amount of the hero worship they currently enjoy from the minority, in exchange for a little more appreciation and respect from the majority, along with a large disposal of the unwarranted distrust that is currently sweeping through this country. It doesn't seem like much to ask for.

And what of the family I spoke about? Sadly, the patient quickly succumbed to his disease two days after I met him; there was no miracle cure to save him from the terminal cancer from which he was suffering. Yet I was told he died in peace, without pain, and with family at his side. Something God would be proud of, no doubt.

Helping Harry

Douglas Olson, MD

ONE WINTER EVENING, I was working at a free clinic in Washington, D.C. I looked at my watch and realized it was 8:30 P.M. I looked out the window. Seeing the streetlight, my mind drifted as I began to imagine my breath turning to steam in the cold night air.

Mr. Harry M. Jacobs was my next patient. Hypertension, diabetes, high cholesterol. He came in every three months. His blood pressure looked good; no complaints today. I got the glucometer to spot-check his blood, grabbed the monofilament line to check for sensation in his feet, and walked in to meet Mr. Jacobs for the first time.

As is typical with my patient interaction, we began by talking about life in general. He told me that he had lived in D.C. for over half his life and that he was a recovering drug user, clean for ten years. His addiction had left him both hepatitis C–positive and with a deep faith in a higher being. He spoke with great candor and openness. And while it would not change anything, I couldn't help but wonder whether he knew that *half* his life was older than my *whole* life.

We talked some more. Lifting his shirt, he showed me his two healed stab wounds and the healed bullet wound that for him defined the 1960s and 1970s. This 59-year-old patient was riveting. And tough. He was not someone who just talked the talk, he walked the walk. His scars were a testament to this. But as we talked some more, he seemed sad about something. With a deep breath, a change in tone, and an expectant state of mind, I asked him about it.

There was a pause. Silence. The kind that you know is no more than five seconds but seems to last for a couple of minutes. The proverbial pin could be heard hitting the floor. And then another one hit. I wanted to ask him whether he heard me but knew he had. His eyes told me so. And before another pin dropped, Harry began to cry in deep, very painful sobs.

He told me that for the past two months, he'd had a steady girlfriend, and for the first time in 20 years, he had begun to love again. He never thought he would! Two days prior, he had come home, and as he got into bed, found a pipe and a little white bag of powder under the mattress. He knew he had to decide between his love and his life. If she stayed, he risked his own ten-year recovery from drugs and alcohol. The decision, he said, was sad and instantaneous. He hadn't spoken to his girlfriend since then.

Harry wasn't depressed, but he had been hurt and was suffering from a devastating loss. He was still saying goodbye to a few weeks of hope, to a rekindled spirit—feelings of passion, concern, and intense emotion for another human being. Harry had long ago buried these feelings, thinking they would be gone forever. And suddenly, without even looking for them, they were exhumed. Suddenly, he was living a life he told me he had only dreamed about. And just as suddenly, that nirvana imploded.

I knew there was nothing I could do. No pharmacy would dispense "time," no matter what I wrote on a prescription pad. I had nothing that could make Harry feel better. No Metformin for his diabetes or hydrochlorothiazide for his blood pressure would help him right now. We both knew this.

I looked him straight in the eye. He looked back. I'm not really sure what he was thinking or feeling. To be honest, I'm not really sure what *I* was thinking or feeling. But I do remember that we connected. I told him I wished there was something I could do for him or say to him that would make him feel a bit better, but that there wasn't. He already knew that. He smiled and wiped the last tear from his eye. His hands still damp with tears, he grabbed my hand, took a deep breath, and simply said, "Thanks."

We went on to talk about his hypertension, diabetes, and the blood that would likely be taken for liver function tests. He had no problems with these conditions, no complaints. He was medication-compliant, was exercising, and was praying and going to church regularly. Harry left that night with some new prescriptions and an appointment for three months later. Nearly a year has passed, but our paths have not crossed again.

Yet Harry remains etched in my mind. More than any other patient, he reminds me that medicine is practiced not to prescribe pills, not to perform surgery, not to conduct research. Harry reminds me that by practicing medicine we have the capacity to restore human dignity. By being human, first and foremost, we can absorb a part of a person's strife and relieve that person of pain. I had done nothing for Harry but admit to him medicine's shortcomings. Even with technology advancing at a dazzling rate, there was nothing we could do to help heal his wounded triad of heart, psyche, and soul.

Harry left the clinic that night after telling his story for the first time to another and after crying for the first time in many years. All I did was listen. Yet that's all he really needed—another human to listen and to be there. No technology can improve that.

Getting Through

Monique Tello, MD, MPH

STANLEY STANISKLAUS WAS dying. Dorothy, the very experienced nurse, had indicated as much by circling her finger downward in the air when he was wheeled into intensive care. I was the resident on call, and I didn't get it.

Dr. Deadpan, the intensive care unit director and my supervisor for the month, translated the gesture: "This man's circling the drain." As he left, he leaned close and whispered, "You'll get it."

Mr. S was a large man, with a large family. Despite a long history of high blood pressure, diabetes, and alcohol abuse, he somehow had never been in the hospital overnight. But a lifetime of bratwurst and beer catches up to anyone. That night, he started throwing up blood—dark, coffee-ground-colored, digested blood. By the time he came to us, he had had a plastic tube in his nose draining the digested blood from him and two intravenous lines dripping pints of transfusion blood into him.

The Stanisklaus clan was in shock. He was their patriarch, magnanimous and indestructible. Every family member had a reason that this could not possibly be happening: "He was fine Sunday! He was eating roast beef and toasting his first great-grandchild's birth! He's clear as a bell and strong as an ox!"

He also reeked of urine, as though it was sweating out of him; the Foley catheter bag was empty. Uh-oh.

But first, we had to deal with this pesky bleeding gut. Dr. Haywood, a kind, gray-haired gastroenterologist, came in and snaked a multipurpose camera into Mr. Stanisklaus. We all saw the swollen veins like evil purple caterpillars crawling up and out of Mr. Stanisklaus's stomach. Varices—these engorged veins were a complication of alcoholism and usually accompanied by liver failure, which he had, in addition to kidney failure.

He was circling.

Dr. Haywood used the scope to cauterize the burst and bleeding vein. The situation was stabilized for the time being. He went to speak to the family in the waiting room, while I went to talk to Mr. S about how sick he was. Mr. S was still sleepy and loopy from the procedure and from his illness.

"Mr. Stanisklaus, do you know where you are?"

He smiled the most sincere and grateful smile, grasping my hand with both of his.

"Thank you, thank you, for all you have done for me. Thank you," he whispered hoarsely.

I sat on the bed and gave him both of my hands. He looked better, pinker from the blood transfusion, smiling from the sedatives.

"Mr. Stanisklaus, we have to talk. Your kidneys are failing. You need to go on a special machine called a dialysis machine, at least for awhile. Do you understand?"

Mr. S started to cry and kept patting and grasping my hands, saying, "Thank you, thanks so much." I smiled, fixed his hair, and watched him. I noticed that his breathing was a bit labored. I glanced up at the monitor. His heart was racing, and his oxygen level was borderline low. This was not good.

"I'm going to go talk to your family," I told him. On my way out I asked the nurse to call for an X-ray, stat.

As I entered the crowded waiting room, the son and daughter jumped up and came forward.

"Hello. I'm Dr. Tello, and I'm the resident doctor in charge of the intensive care unit tonight. I know you've met many doctors today, and I am sorry that you're meeting one more, but I will be with your father all night and most of tomorrow." I was about to say how worried I was for him, then launch into an explanation of kidney failure and dialysis. I had planned it all out.

But the son blurted, "When can he go home?"

I looked around at the whole clan, and not one face registered the surprise I felt upon hearing his question. I must have looked bewildered.

The son's eyes narrowed. "The gastroenterologist just came out here and told us that he had fixed the bleeding vein. That was the problem, right? So we want to know when we can take Dad home. We don't want anything . . . bad . . . to happen to him here in the hospital."

I am a petite woman, and I look young for my age, which in this business does not inspire immediate confidence. That night had been busy, and my white coat was stained with coffee and pen marks. My nails were bitten to the quick. I thought: Who doesn't want the kindly, experienced gray-haired physician? Who wants a young, frazzled doctor-in-training?

I tucked my hands in my whitish coat pockets. "Let's sit down," I said, trying to look composed and act in charge. "The bleeding vein isn't the only problem. Your father is so, so sick. His kidneys and liver are failing. He's having trouble breathing, and I just ordered a chest X-ray."

"What do you mean? Look, is Dr. Haywood still here? No offense, but he really seemed to know what he was talking about." The son glanced at his sister for support. The whole family nodded.

She stepped forward. "Can we see our father at least, while you go and get someone more senior to talk to us?"

I felt a blush creep over me; this was familiar. I acquiesced, of course. "The nurses don't like more than three or four family members at a time, so why don't you choose and then let's go in?"

The daughter crossed her arms over her chest. "They let *all* of us in the hospital room before." Even the teenagers in the group were rolling their eyes and making outraged snorting noises, as they probably did with their parents sometimes.

"Fine; if the nurses have a problem, they'll let you know." I smiled tightly and swiped my badge to let everyone into Mr. S's room.

I called Dr. Deadpan and tried not to sound desperate.

"You can handle this," he said. "You'll get it." He gave some medical guidance and hung up.

I called the nephrologist. I told him that I thought the shortness of breath was due to kidney failure, that fluid was building up in Mr. S's lungs.

"Give him some Lasix; see if it helps. Call me if it doesn't work," he said. Lasix is a diuretic, and it makes people urinate extra fluid, if they can still urinate. Really, I had just wanted him to come in, to face this tough crowd for me.

But no one was going to come in.

Meanwhile, the chest X-ray hadn't been taken and Mr. S was struggling to breathe. His oxygen levels dropped below normal. Dorothy the nurse pushed past all the family members and placed an oxygen cannula in Mr. S's nose.

"He's never needed oxygen before. What in hell is going on?" the daughter hissed at me in the hallway.

I nodded, trying to convey understanding and concern. "We're waiting for a chest X-ray, but let me get in there and examine him."

"We're staying in the room; we're not leaving."

I took a deep breath and entered the small room. Everyone went quiet, as if they'd been talking about me. I placed my stethoscope on Mr. S's chest. He again took my hand and smiled. I laughed, and it came out like a grateful sob.

"Thank you, thank you," he said.

"No, thank *you*," I replied. I meant it. Though I knew he was confused, his sincere acceptance of me gave me strength.

His lungs sounded crackly. I turned to face the family. "He's putting more fluid on his lungs. We're going to give some medicine to clear it and get some tests of the heart."

"What?" the sister spoke, her face mean. "You come in and listen to him for three seconds, and then you want to give him medicine? Didn't you just say you were going to get an X-ray? I'm just not sure you know what you're doing."

Though she spoke quietly, she was taller than me, and had her arms crossed, and I felt very small.

Suddenly an alarm sounded from the monitor. Dorothy leapt up. "Brady down to 40." Mr. S's heart rate was dropping rapidly. In the space of three seconds his eyes glazed over, his skin tinged blue, and he fell limp.

My own heart stopped. "Okay, call a code, now." I grabbed the panicked sister's shoulder, hard, pushed her toward the door, and said, "His heart's failing. You just have to trust me, please. We'll do everything we can." She and the rest of the family moved like a herd of cats into the waiting room, suspicious glances turning to panic as the code alarm sounded. All over the hospital, the speakers were blaring "Code 3, Medical ICU, Code 3, Medical ICU" over and over again. Any and all residents, respiratory therapists, and anesthesiologists still in the hospital were summoned to that room stat. They ran past the S family through the double doors of the ICU, some shouldering through like football players, others striding in grimly. Every time the doors opened, I could see the straining faces of Mr. S's entire family.

I called out orders by rote. "Bag him, turn up the O_2 all the way. Let's get him on a board. Get the code cart here. Can I have 1 milligram of atropine? Get some epi ready . . . Set up to intubate . . . "

I gazed with great expectation at the cardiac monitor. The heart rate slowly increased. Mr. S was intubated and put on a respirator. His color returned.

The EKG and labs told the tale: the strain of the massive bleed had triggered a heart attack. This, followed by heavy transfusions, caused heart failure. There was still fluid on his lungs, but positive pressure from the respirator kept the lungs inflated and oxygenating. With his very recent bleed and his concomitant kidney and liver failure, we were very limited in what we could give him. But his heart rate and blood pressure recovered somewhat.

"I should get the cardiologist in here now," I said, and left to make the call.

A sleepy cardiologist answered; I knew him, and he was exactly the experienced doctor whose backup I could really use.

"Wow, we're stuck between a rock and a hard place with this one," he said. "I'm not sure what I can offer at this point. Doesn't sound like a thrombosis issue, sounds like it was a perfusion issue, and you've got that under control. Why don't you see how things go and keep me updated?"

He was not going to come in either.

I called Dr. Deadpan and the nephrologist and got more of the same.

And I thought: They're right.

I marched to the waiting room with a feeling of impending doom. I realized the family must have watched the code team run in and file out, and I wasn't sure whether they'd been given any information. They must have been tortured.

They fell on me. "How is he?"

"He's alive," I said. There was a palpable, collective gasp of relief.

"What happened?" asked the daughter.

I took a deep breath. "Well, that stomach bleed put his body over the edge. He lost a lot of blood really fast and got a lot of fluids and transfusions really fast, which is hard on any body. He had a heart attack and is in heart failure. This, plus the kidney and liver failure and the recent bleed leaves us very few options for treatment."

"What are you saying?" asked the son.

I just kept going. "If he goes unstable again, if anything else happens, there isn't much we can do. And I've spoken to quite a few senior docs about this." I scanned their faces, pleading in my mind: *Believe me, there is nothing else anyone can do.*

The faces were still so angry. "Can we see him now, please?" asked the daughter.

"Of course."

The whole family piled into the ICU. There were sharp gasps and moans when they saw him. His face was puffy. He had a new, large intravenous line taking up the whole right side of his neck. He had a breathing tube in his mouth and was hooked up to a respirator. He had more intravenous lines in his swollen arms. He was bruised and bloodied and bandaged.

Then the daughter grabbed my elbow. "Come out into the hallway with me now," she demanded. "Our father came in here with a bleeding vein and it was fixed. Now he's falling apart. And you're, like, this little student doctor. I don't want you doing anything else, and I mean *anything else*, to MY father, at all." She spat out the last sentence.

A few other family members drifted out, murmuring quietly. Although I couldn't see them, I could sense that everyone in the ICU stopped what they were doing to watch the drama, this resident lynching.

But by some miracle, no tears welled up in me and spilled over into that ICU hallway. What welled up were all the times I'd walked into a patient's hospital room, only to be mistaken for the physical therapist, social worker, or cafeteria tray collector; and all the times I smiled and said nothing, not only because I knew those roles were important but mostly because I didn't have the guts to assert myself. For years I learned to anticipate "but you look so young to be a doctor," to tolerate the occasional "but you're too cute to be a doctor," to recognize the wary look or questioning tone of voice, and to back down. I learned to qualify my statements, to offer to get "a more senior opinion." I learned to call the old gray-haired guys in for backup, and I did so often, and the cycle continued.

But tonight I was high and dry and, somehow, sure that I was right. All the unexpressed outrage puffed me up and pushed me forward with a deep breath, resident breath reeking of a full 16 hours of consuming nothing more than a large Dunkin' Donuts coffee. Maybe that's what made the daughter step back. But as she did, I moved forward, and then kept going, little step by little step, each word direct and clear and calm, coming from somewhere within me:

"Look, I don't know what your family dynamics are and what kind of denial you're in, but your father is dying and that's pretty obvious to everyone. I'm pulling out the stops to keep his broken body going, and you are making my job VERY difficult. There are no other doctors coming in because I AM the doctor. There is a very good chance that your father will die tonight. I am telling you, if that is the case, there is nothing that I would have done to cause it, and there is nothing that anyone can do to prevent it. There are not many doctors who would have put up with the disrespect you have shown me tonight. Let me be clear, I am not here for you. I am here for the man in that room who thanked me with his tears. You got it?"

As soon as the words were out of my mouth, I wondered where on earth they had come from, and how I could put them back.

She stared at me in utter silence. The nurses stared at me in utter silence.

I was shocked as much by what I didn't say as by what I said. There was no profanity, as much as I wanted to add a "you bitch" in there. Both the outburst and my restraint left me absolutely paralyzed, unable to anticipate her reaction or my response.

I thought of two cats posturing before a fight.

Then the daughter lowered her eyes and lifted her hands to her face. She started to sob.

"It's just that he was fine yesterday . . . " Her brother put his arm around her.

I felt as if we had just crossed the equator, as though the magnetic fields surrounding us had shifted.

And then the alarms went off again.

"Brady down . . . Asystole," called the nurse.

The family was ushered out and the code game played out again . . . and again. Three times Mr. S's heart stopped, and three times he was brought back with brutal pounding and the strongest medications.

The third time, one of the nurses exclaimed, "This is hopeless, we're torturing this man," just loud enough for the family, still out in the waiting room, to hear. I could tell they had heard, as I glanced up and met their haggard stares.

The daughter stood up and waved her arms in the air, yelling, "NO MORE, PLEASE, please, no more," before she collapsed back down, sobbing.

The last thing I wanted was to interact with the family I had hurt in the midst of the most difficult experience of their family life. But I had to. As kindly as possible, I told the truth: "Listen, his heart is tired, it just wants to stop beating. There is nothing else we can do. We can let him rest now." And the whole group nodded and cried. I offered to let them be with him, and the wonderful ICU staff ushered people in and handed out Kleenex. Soon, the monitor blips slowed to the drone of asystole, as Dorothy discreetly turned down the volume.

I retreated to a back table and sat down. I had Mr. S's chart in front of me, and I stared at it and wrote nothing. I sat until after the family had been advised about chaplains and funeral homes and left, and the nurses opened the room's only window, as is customary, allowing the soul to float out.

I tiptoed in and pronounced him, though there was no need. The curtains were pulled, the room darkened. His eyes were already closed, the tubes removed from his nose and mouth, his skin the color of split eggplant. I took his cool hand and whispered, "Thank you, for all you have done for me, thank you."

NIGHT IN THE EMERGENCY ROOM

Bryan Bordeaux, DO, MPH

IT WAS A misty early Thursday evening in late March, and surprisingly warm for that time of year. The snow was melting fast. I was staffing the emergency room that night, like I normally did for a handful of shifts each month, and was expecting it to be slow. The rural Appalachian hospital I was working in had 22 beds and an emergency room consisting of four stretchers separated by curtains.

As usual, I had worked a full day in the office beforehand, seeing mainly complex, elderly patients. As part of my pre-ER ritual, I left the office at 4:30, drove the windy eight miles into town, purchased a six-inch buffalo chicken sub on whole wheat, and ate my dinner in the on-call room before my shift officially started at 5:00.

I watched a few minutes of local TV in the constricted, cinderblock-walled room from a creaky hospital bed that doubled as a sofa, before being called to evaluate an out-of-town visitor with lower abdominal pain. In her mid-40s, she was twisting from side to side to get comfortable. After a brief introduction, I asked her to tell me what had happened. She said that for the past couple of days she had been having some pain in the lower left side of her groin that had gotten progressively worse throughout the day, to the point now where she was nauseous and had vomited before arrival. "I've also had a fever and my skin has been red and painful in the area," she explained.

When I lifted her gown to examine her abdomen, the diagnosis was immediately clear: she had a large strangulated hernia. In other words, a portion of her intestines was trapped in the gap of her abdominal wall. The blood supply to the intestine was cut off, and the restricted portion of bowel had begun to die. Normal bacteria from inside her gut had begun to leak out from the dead tissue and led to an infection in the surrounding area. This was a surgical emergency, but unfortunately, we did not have a surgeon available. There was about a year between the time that our own surgeon had left the hospital and when the surgeons from Towanda started covering our emergency department. I had no choice but to call an ambulance and transfer the patient to a nearby hospital so that she could have surgery that evening.

I immediately called that hospital's emergency department (ED), located 45 minutes away, and spoke to a very friendly physician there who readily agreed to accept the patient in transfer. We notified the ambulance dispatcher, who sent one of the county's two ambulance crews up to our hospital.

There was a hitch. The patient's health insurance was from an out-of-state company and she would need to get pre-approval for her hospital visit, or else she might have to pay for the surgery and all of the associated costs, which could be many thousands of dollars. Unfortunately, the hospital in Scranton was not an approved facility, but the smaller one in Towanda was. We called the ED there and I spoke to the surgeon on call, who agreed to see the patient. She called her insurance company from the gurney to confirm that her care would be covered, and when it was, she allowed us to transfer her. We called back the ED in Scranton and the ambulance crew.

Before she left the building, another patient arrived in the emergency room. He was a man in his late 50s who filled the air with Old Milwaukee Light and a limited selection of loud and repeated profanities. He had slipped on the ice about an hour before and literally dragged himself into our hospital. His swollen left foot dangled loose and lifeless from the rest of the leg. A quick X-ray confirmed that he had fractured both his tibia and fibula. I could not feel a pulse in his foot, and he also needed emergency surgery. No X-ray was required to determine whether his left ankle was broken; his swollen and bruised foot wobbled from side to side when he lifted his leg. I got an X-ray to evaluate the extent of the damage. As we all expected, both of his lower leg bones, the tibia and fibula, were sheared off and not aligned at all. Of even greater concern, his foot was cold and I knew that blood flow was compromised, because I could not feel pulses and his foot did not blanch and pink up within a few seconds when pressed by my finger, a physical sign called capillary refill.

I called our orthopedist, who mainly worked a half hour away but who came to our hospital each Wednesday to see patients. He was always accessible but often a bit gruff. He spoke fast, with a rhythmic accent: "Yeah, this man needs surgery tonight. Send him down to our emergency room and I'll see him." Click. When I explained the situation to the patient, he immediately refused, saying, "I want to go home. I am not going to Towanda. Just give me some pain medications and I'll be all right." He cursed at me over and over again, and I did my best to maintain a professional tone. He kept insisting that he did not need to be transferred, but when pressed further, his reason was disclosed with sadness and shame: "I don't have health insurance. I cannot afford to take an ambulance and I cannot pay for the surgery. I'll get by."

I suspected that, like many people suffering from addiction, he was more interested in getting buzzed that evening than receiving the care he needed. It was only after ten minutes of my insisting that emergency surgery was the only way to save his foot from amputation that he admitted that he did not have health insurance and was afraid of the bills associated with his care. He grudgingly agreed to be transferred, after I assured him that there were government and charity programs available that might be able to cover most of his medical expenses. We called the second ambulance crew, and within a half hour he was strapped on the stretcher, cursing as he went out the door.

By now, it was around 7:30, and I thought I might have a break for a while. I was starting to complete my paperwork when the ED phone rang again. A mother was coming in with her sick child. They would be there in about five minutes. I took a deep breath—there was a reason I went into internal medicine and not family practice or pediatrics. I felt a little more comfortable caring for children than when I started, but unless they had something really simple like an ear infection or the common cold, I felt uneasy.

As the parents carried their infant daughter down the long hallway where I was waiting, I noticed two things about the baby: she was very small and very limp. The overweight mother was 25, with plain features, and her husband was a year or two older, but his lanky frame and boyish face made him look 15. Their daughter appeared to be the size and weight of the six-inch sub I had for dinner that evening.

The patient was born at 28 weeks and had been in the neonatal intensive care unit at a major hospital for another 12 weeks until her estimated due date. She had been discharged from that hospital about a week ago, and the parents informed me that she had not been feeding at all for three days and had been spitting up some of her food for a day or two before that.

I thought to myself, "Oh God, why me?" As an internist, I was trained to treat adults, not children. Most of the patients in the ER were adults, and the children who came in were almost always school age and had minor complaints like an earache, rash, or injured limb. Still, I had no choice in this underserved community but to treat all comers as best I could. I'd become more comfortable over time with older children, but I always feared a sick newborn.

My palms and soles started to sweat and I could feel my heart throbbing. It was one of those times in your life when you feel a rare mixture of fear and lucid poise. I had no idea what this child had, but it was something serious, and I was not sufficiently trained and our hospital was not adequately equipped to diagnose or treat it. My mind flashed back to my pediatrics training as a medical student. Could it be an intestinal infection or blockage? Meningitis? Pneumonia? How could I even tell what she had? All I knew was that this child needed to be somewhere else. And she should have been there 24 hours ago.

I performed a very brief and focused exam. The infant lay still and quiet on the exam table. This was the first baby I had ever examined who did not resist at all. Her skin was dry and she had poor capillary refill on her arms and legs, a sign that she was severely dehydrated.

I weighed the pros and cons of trying to get some fluids into her versus immediate transfer. Because of her size and dehydration, a traditional IV was not possible and she would need an intraosseous catheter placed. This requires that the provider use a T-shaped device to repeatedly twist a hollow metal screw into a child's leg until it reached the bone marrow, where fluids could be infused. Despite the relative simplicity of the procedure (or so it is said in Pediatric Advanced Life Support), I froze at the idea.

Usually when caring for a patient, I am able to detach myself enough from an emergency situation and work almost automatically. In this case, however, I had never done the procedure before and thought about manually drilling into the child's leg with a screw. Would I create any long-term damage to the bone and thereby affect her ability to live a normal life? Would there be a big scar as she aged? If the procedure was really not necessary and I harmed the girl, would the parents sue me? On the other hand, if she died of dehydration because of my inaction, that would be infinitely worse. Because I expected a rapid transfer and am not very good with my hands (with patients or around the house), I chose against placing the intraosseous catheter.

To begin the transfer process, I called back the hospital where I had transferred the woman with the hernia and spoke to the same emergency room physician. I prayed that he would be able to help again, since I often had difficulty with transfers to another hospital no matter how sick the patient. This time he refused to take the patient because their pediatricians did not treat children so young and fragile. He recommended that I try to transfer her back to the hospital where she was born and initially treated after birth. It was a larger hospital but a two-hour drive. Just then, Michelle, one of the nurses from the hospital, wandered by and said to the mother, "Hi, Jenn, I heard that you were coming in to have your daughter evaluated." She glanced toward the baby, who was about six feet away and beside me. "She looks fine to me—I'd just give her some Tylenol and she'll be okay. Probably just a bug that's been going around." She then explained to me that the mother used to clean her home.

After she left, I explained to the parents again that I thought there was something seriously wrong with their daughter and we needed to transfer her quickly. By then, it was 8:15 P.M.

Because I did not know whether she would survive the long drive, I suggested to the parents that we try to transfer her to another nearby hospital more specialized in pediatric care. It was also 45 minutes away, but unlike the other hospitals, was in a neighboring state. The parents explained to me that they were insured through an HMO that only had contracts with hospitals in our state.

Without any other options, I called the out-of-state hospital and spoke to their emergency department doctor, who was very understanding and eager to help. He directed me to their ambulance dispatcher, who assured me that they had a helicopter flight crew available and ready to come to our rescue. Ten minutes later, after a confirmation call, everything was set: the crew would fly out and be at our hospital in 20 minutes. I was not sure who was more overjoyed with the news, the parents or me.

As I began to complete the transfer paperwork, the phone rang. It was the helicopter crew changing their plans because they were grounded by fog. I went back to the family with this devastating news. They must have seen the frustration in my eyes but remained calm. The best thing we could do now was to see if there was a county ambulance available to race the patient to this distant hospital. It was 9:00, and the child was lying nearly lifeless, like a plastic doll.

The dispatcher said that both ambulances I had sent were still out on assignments and she expected that they could have a crew at our hospital a little after 10:00. I snapped back at her that this was unacceptable, if only to vent my frustration. She calmly but firmly reiterated that she had nothing else to offer. Now worried that this flaccid newborn child was going to die in front of us, I reconsidered placing the catheter. While weighing my options one last time, I took a wide plastic pen out of my lapel pocket and flexed it between my fingers, clenched my teeth, and shuffled around the hallway, angrily mumbling.

The parents came back to me with their daughter and belongings in hand, insisting that they could not wait any longer and were going to drive her to the large hospital themselves. This was not an option I was considering, but I realized that it was probably the best way to try to save her life.

As they raced out the door, I chased after them and asked that they call me with an update after she was seen at the other hospital. They did not call that evening. Days passed and there was still no word from them. I was convinced that she had died in their car in the backwoods and they were already talking to their lawyer while still grieving. I was afraid to call them but needed to know what happened. Eight days later, they called and told me that she had a congenital narrowing in her stomach called pyloric stenosis, had surgery to repair it, and was doing just fine back at home. I could finally put that long night behind me.

Angel of Mercy, Angel of Death

Monique Tello, MD, MPH

SHE COULD NOT speak, walk, eat, or even breathe, and she would not die. So we killed her.

I had known her only three weeks. Those three weeks working in the intensive care unit seemed like months, even years, of gut-twisting cardiac arrest codes, hovering over the dead and dying, late-night calls to family members, seeing and causing human anguish. There were no limits on medical residents' work hours yet. We were there at dawn every day and then overnight every third night. The overnight shifts started at dawn and ended when the work was done, late afternoon or evening the next day. I was falling asleep at stoplights and had insomnia when I got home.

But I sure was glad that I wasn't Mrs. N.

Mrs. N had shown up in the emergency room three months before, gasping, her lips and fingertips tinged blue. The savvy ER doc threaded a breathing tube down her windpipe, and she was hooked up to a ventilator and delivered to the intensive care unit, diagnosed with chronic blood clots to the lungs and heart failure. She had gone into shock and part of her gut had choked off, died, and rotted inside her. She went to the operating room twice. She had more complications, kidney failure and liver failure and abscesses, and more procedures, a pacemaker placement for slow heart rate, antibiotics, experimental medicines. She developed a bedsore, skin that dies from the constant pressure of lying in bed day after day. The surgeons had to cut and scrape off the dead tissue many times, until her lower back and buttocks were ragged beef jerky that oozed yellow fluid. The germs in the open wound had a party with the antibiotics and developed resistance, so she was colonized with all the dreaded superbugs that no one wants to spread around. Her heart and lungs continued to fail, and her medications list and ventilator setting were increasing daily.

Mrs. N had had a tracheostomy after the first few weeks, and the breathing tube was sticking out of her neck, attached to the machine. Every morning, as a ritual, I would don the requisite yellow paper gown and gloves and mask and inhale deeply in the hallway. I would knock gently and push open the door and no matter what, I would be greeted with the stench of her wound and germs. She could not talk, but every morning when I went in the room and held her hand, she smiled.

Mrs. N was awake. She smiled, and sometimes she cried. She smiled at the nurses when they changed her colostomy bag or sponged her clean, at anyone who touched her softly or spoke kind words. She cried silent tears when she was rolled, when the bed was changed, when the surgeons came to check her wound, when anyone asked her a question.

Her husband scowled.

He was a constant; as long as security would let him in, he was there. He would sit next to her and hold her hand and stroke her hair, would tell her stories and then bark at the nurses, shoo the doctors. When I walked in my first morning, he stood up and blocked me.

"Who are you? What's your rank?" he demanded. Mr. N was a diminutive man with a beard and cane, very ex-military and very suspicious. I had been warned.

"Good morning, I'm Dr. Tello," I said, and I shook his hand. "I graduated from medical school in 2001, and I am a first-year resident here. I'll be helping out with your wife's care for the month. I'm the person on the medical team who will be coming in every day and checking on your wife. And I'll always ask you what you think and give you the team's assessment."

He had stood leaning on his cane, staring at me, measuring me. He refused to wear the gown and gloves that everyone else wore. Everyone had given up on making him garb. He stood and scowled at me for what seemed like a full minute. I did not look away.

He put his head down, thoughtful. Finally he nodded his assent and sat down. After that, every morning he would stand as I entered as if to block my path and only backed down when I greeted him and he had taken his measure of me.

One morning as I entered, he stood up angrily and said, "She's in pain. She needs more pain medicines." I looked over to Mrs. N. She looked over at me and smiled.

"What hurts, ma'am, what's bothering you?" I asked, but she seemed confused and only fluttered her hands weakly by her sides. She never mouthed any words to anyone; she wouldn't use a blinking system or point to words on a card. We thought she had suffered a large stroke early on in the hospital course, when her blood pressure was so low for so many days and there probably wasn't enough blood and oxygen going to the brain. It was almost impossible to tell for sure, as she could not have an MRI of the brain, due to her pacemaker. Neurologists and psychologists had seen her and said she had an expressive aphasia, which meant that she couldn't communicate what she was thinking to us. She had no voice for us. We didn't know how much she understood. Questions made her upset.

And my question to her that morning made her upset, made her eyes fill with tears, and she looked over to her husband as if to ask him something.

"See? She has pain; you need to give her something for the pain." He made his way haltingly over to the side of the bed, and I saw that he was limping more than usual and holding his right hip.

"Sir, are you all right?" I asked.

He looked up at me with surprise. "I'm fine. I have arthritis. I'm fine because I take my pain medication. Will you do your job and get her some pain medication please?"

I stood quietly for a moment, then examined Mrs. N. Her gray hair was combed to one side. Her breath was minty from the sponge soaked in mouthwash that her husband applied every morning; he would hold it to her lips and let her suckle at it, let her enjoy the cold moisture, the only thing that went in her mouth. She was fed through an intravenous line; what was left of her intestines could not function.

Her neck was obscured by the bandages covering her large intravenous line and more bandages covering the tracheostomy hole in her neck where the breathing tube went in. Her chest was covered with cardiac monitoring leads. I found a space and listened to her heart with its whooshes and gurgles, and I could feel the pacemaker through the skin of her chest. I pulled the sheets up to cover her groin and pulled her gown up to reveal her stomach, a knotted mass of healing scars, the colostomy contraption and bag filled with liquid stool. I put all this back and then pulled aside the sheets over her legs to check her legs, enveloped in inflatable plastic wrap that puffed up and then deflated every few minutes to help prevent blood clots.

There was so little of her left to examine. Then I saw her toes. They were painted seashell pink.

"Oh!" I exclaimed. "This is new!"

Mr. N looked down and flushed a deep scarlet.

"She used to like to paint her nails. I can't do her fingers because of the oxygen monitors"—the little probe that clips on to the finger to measure the oxygen—"so I painted her toes instead. Just last night."

"Well. That's very nice." I leaned in to Mrs. N. "Your toes look very nice," I said, and I smiled and patted her hand, and she smiled.

I left the room and pulled off the gown and gloves and sat down to write my note in the chart.

"I can't stand those beady little eyes." Lisette the nurse slammed one of the volumes of the chart onto the conference table. "He's evil is what he is, he's a control freak and he likes it that she's helpless and hurting." There were murmurs of assent from the staff gathered, charting toward the end of their night shift.

"Someone should talk to that man, talk him into letting his poor wife go," said another nurse, and I felt a few eyes shift over to me.

Residents on the case had first approached Mr. N about home hospice after her first month in the hospital. Her condition was deemed terminal and her quality of life poor, and it seemed a reasonable option. He had yelled and thrown things:

"No, no, and no! I won't kill my wife, and I won't let you kill her either."

Attendings had sat down with him "to discuss options." The answer was no.

A few times Mr. N had grumbled and mumbled while I was in the room, "Doctors nowadays don't want to take care of patients. It's all about the bottom line. No one really cares anymore."

And every day the wound festered.

I was on a Friday-night overnight call toward the end of my month when one of the nurses asked me to speak to Mr. N again about "code status." There were seven medical beds; all full, all stable. We needed a bed. She was taking a bed. And what for? What were we doing for her?

"It is a hopeless case," she said. "That husband is not living in reality; he sees her as she was, not how she is. We have to make him see." She leaned forward. "*You* can make him see. He trusts you. You can get her to a Code C." This means hospice and a comfortable, inevitable death.

I knew this. I had been thinking about it every time I walked into the room with my breath held, every time the surgeons came to change the wound-vacuum and needed my help, every time we went up on her ventilator settings. Mrs. N was never going to be stable enough to leave the ICU, and she was never going to die there, either. It was her purgatory, and we were there with her.

The next week, her daughter came to visit. I had been told she was coming, and I knew from Mr. N's mumbling that she was "obstinate and independent."

I had a plan.

The daughter, Nancy, was blond and willowy, dressed smart, a business lady. She shone with brisk practicality. She lived on the West Coast; she hadn't been home since the first months of her mother's admission. Mr. N went to a doctor's appointment, and Nancy sat with her mother. I wanted her to be there for the wound-vacuum change.

I watched her face as the surgery resident turned off the suction and peeled back the wet, warm foam padding. The gaping wound of Mrs. N's buttocks was raw, jagged, and pinkish, oozing blood. There was some granulation tissue, I noted. It certainly looked better now than it had at the beginning of the month. But it still smelled, a warm, meaty, digestive smell. Nancy's hand went to her mouth and she disguised her retch with a small cough.

"My God," she whispered, choking.

I steered her out of the room and into the hallway.

"My God!" She held both manicured hands over her stomach. "Can they . . . fix that? Will that ever heal?"

"Well, it's not likely," I answered. "There hasn't been much improvement in this many months. You need lots of energy and good health to heal, and your mother has irreversible heart and lung problems, and with the liver failing from the artificial nutrition she gets through the IV line, we're not sure how long we can keep up."

"But what are the chances of her getting out of the hospital? Of going home and living out the rest of her life?"

I searched her eyes, knowing full well that Mr. N had been feeding her optimistic lies for several months now. "It's not likely that your mother will ever be discharged from this intensive care unit. Her prognosis is very poor. We would even say that she is terminal."

Though I kept my voice soft and sorry, and though Nancy remained standing, I could tell from her eyes that the effect of my words on her was that of a club on a baby seal.

Nancy's hands fluttered to her mouth and she looked away. She took a few deep breaths, then turned back to me. "Does he know? Does my father know how bad it is?"

I held her gaze for a few seconds. "Several of the head doctors have tried to speak with him about hospice, about letting your mother go. He has not been receptive to the idea."

She let out a small sound, like an "Oh" or a "No," and leaned against the wall.

I waited.

"I'll need to discuss this with him and maybe . . . with some of the more . . . senior doctors, if you don't mind . . ."

"Of course, that's absolutely understandable. I can make the arrangements."

She seemed deflated. I felt a pang of guilt, seeing in her some of Mrs. N's unfailing smile. I imagined Nancy's long trip here and long hours at home with that man. The man who painted his dying wife's toenails seashell pink.

I leaned over and placed my hand on Nancy's forearm. "Are you okay?" I whispered.

"No, I'm fine. I knew. I just didn't want to know." And she walked out of the intensive care unit, tall and determined.

The next day, Lisette the nurse came up to me. "The daughter wants to talk with you," she said, smiling, congratulating.

I arranged a meeting with her, Mr. N, and the ICU attending physician. We sat in the uncomfortable plastic chairs of the dingy resident's teaching room, as there was no family room. There was a chalkboard with the diagnostic algorithm for pulmonary embolism written out, what made the diagnosis high probability, low probability, indeterminate. There were "interesting EKGs" pinned to the board. The trash can was overflowing with fast-food wrappers, and there were no windows. Nancy sat tall and pert in her chair; Mr. N looked deflated, looking down at his hands on his lap. The attending looked at me, as if to indicate that this was my show. I began:

"I understand you'd like to consider hospice care."

There was quiet nodding. Mr. N continued to look down. I met Nancy's eyes.

"We can start by making your mother more comfortable with some pain medication, and then we can remove the breathing machine. You can be there then or come in after we've disconnected it."

There was a pause. Mr. N's mouth twitched and his hands shook, but he did not speak.

Nancy spoke: "How long will it take?"

I glanced over at my attending. He gave an impercep-
tible shrug.

I guessed. "It's hard to say, but I think you can prepare
to be here for at least a few hours."

There was quiet, and then Mr. N whispered, "I wish
we knew what she wanted."

Nancy did not look at him but did incline her head in
his direction. "Dad, she would not want to live like this.
This is not living. We're doing the right thing for her."

She waited.

Mr. N nodded.

"Would you like to speak to the chaplain?" I offered.

At the same time:

"Yes," said Nancy.

"No," said Mr. N.

A space.

I looked at Nancy. "A chaplain will be available if you
wish."

There was a movement at the door. It was the head
nurse with some pamphlets. They were wasting no time. I
added, "The nurses are here with some information, some
logistical information. I'm sure you have questions . . . "
I left to others all the discussion on last rites, visitors, sitting with her, the morgue, the funeral home, the services.
I escaped as well as I could, with a nod and a curt smile.
The attending beat me to the door.

The arrangements were made, a quiet buzzing about
the periphery of the ICU. I ran around playing doctor for

the other patients, but I was closely following the movements of the nurses, the chaplain, the social worker, and all the support staff. I kept catching fragments of conversation: "They're really going to do it today." "Finally, what a blessing!" "The daughter talked some sense into him."

Some other family members gathered; I recognized some of them and tried not to make eye contact for fear I'd be drawn into a lengthy discussion. They went into the room with Nancy and Mr. N. I kept glancing at the closed door, afraid they would emerge and announce that they had changed their minds, that the torture of Mrs. N would continue, at their bidding and at my hands.

Finally, the door opened. Mr. N seemed confused, unsure where to direct his steps. But Nancy put her hand on her father's shoulder and said to me, "We'll be in the waiting room. Please come get us as soon as the machines are disconnected." The whole family trailed out. The desk nurse had buzzed the ICU door open for them. Staff cleared out of their way. Then all eyes turned to me and Lisette. The respiratory therapist had been waiting with us, and he now stood up as well. I realized then that everyone had been holding their breath, waiting for the family to either go through with this or change their minds.

"Gown up, and let's do this," said Lisette.

Mrs N was awake, staring at the framed photograph on the windowsill. "How are you, ma'am?" asked Lisette. Mrs. N nodded and smiled as always. She seemed more tired somehow, as if the edges of her eyes were drawn down in spite of the smile, and it made her seem sad. Was she sad?

Lisette sat on the edge of the bed. "Let me explain. We're going to unhook this tube from you now. You won't feel any pain. All right?"

Mrs. N looked up at Lisette, smiling. Then she seemed to recognize her, and her look changed; her eyes smiled, and the effect was one of trust.

I tried to stay out of Mrs. N's view. I folded my hands in front of me, and I noticed that I was sweating, heart pounding, feeling a little woozy. Lisette hung a bag of clear medicine to the pole and hooked it into her line. The bag read "MSO_4"—morphine. When people are dying from not being able to breathe, a little morphine takes away the agony, the drowning sensation. Lisette let a small dose run into the line, then slowed it to a drip.

She nodded to the respiratory therapist. The respiratory therapist flicked off the breathing machine and then unhooked the tube from the tracheostomy. Lisette straightened out the bandages and the sheets and we all watched Mrs. N breathe.

She was breathing on her own. I looked at Lisette. She looked at me. We both looked at the respiratory therapist. The feeling I had not allowed myself to feel hit me now in waves of doubt and self-recrimination. I felt like I was suffocating. What were we doing?

Then Mrs. N coughed and sputtered a bit, and her brow furrowed.

I breathed deeply.

"Let me suction her," said the respiratory therapist, and he used the suction device to clear out the tracheostomy. Great green plugs of mucus were sucked into the device and into the trap.

Mrs. N's breathing came faster now, and she looked worried, panicked. She rolled her head weakly to the side and looked at Lisette with questions in her eyes. She looked as though she had no real understanding of what was happening but trusted us and trusted that we meant her no harm.

I felt as if I might vomit.

Lisette leaned in very close to Mrs. N. "It's all right, ma'am, it's going to be all right," she said, and she stroked the woman's forehead. The respiratory therapist was busy packing up equipment and making his way out the door. I watched Mrs. N and saw that her eyes were beginning to flutter.

Then I noticed that Lisette's free hand was on the morphine pump, and that it was running, running at maximum speed. The morphine was in a 250-milliliter bag, mixed so that it was 1 milligram of morphine per 1 milliliter. I watched the numbers on the pump; the morphine was running in at maximum, and the seconds ticked by.

I watched Lisette stroking Mrs. N's head and smiling at her, cooing at her softly. Mrs. N was falling asleep. Her breathing was coming slower, slower.

"Lisette," I whispered.

"Lisette," my voice broke.

She looked up across the bed at me and there was no guise, no malice, only explanation. "Just a little morphine bolus, to take the edge off." Then down again to Mrs. N. "You'll be okay, ma'am, you'll be okay." She never stopped smiling or stroking Mrs. N's head.

I stood and did nothing but feel awful.

Lisette turned the pump back down to a drip. Mrs. N now lay sleeping, breath soft, a slight gurgle from the mucus in the tracheostomy tube.

Lisette's face was calm, no challenge. I saw that she was doing what she thought was absolutely correct. She spent more time with Mrs. N than I did. I had talked the family into this decision; I had studied them and pushed them to the Code C. I had no right to object.

But I objected, silently.

Out loud I said, "I'll get the family."

"I'll stay here," said Lisette.

I hesitated just a second.

But I had made my decision also. I walked out and into the waiting room. They were there, and my face must have held some kind of horror, because they all blanched at seeing me.

"Come on; I'll be honest, there's not much time," I said. I ushered them back into the room and followed. We made no pretense at gowns and gloves now.

Mrs. N breathed for another two or three minutes, and Lisette duly suctioned her. She had placed an oxygen mask over her tracheostomy tube. She had arranged her hair the way Mr. N usually did.

When she breathed her last breath, Mr. N put his head on her chest and sobbed. Lisette and I left the room, leaving the family to mourn. I had an overwhelming desire to wash my hands. I wanted a shower. Instead, one of the nurses clapped me on the shoulder.

"God bless you, Doctor. Thank God that woman has some peace."

Another staff member nearby commented, "You played that son-of-a-bitch like a violin. Good work."

The unit desk secretary handed me a stack of papers. "The death certificate. The body release. Et cetera. Have fun," she droned.

I sat down with the paperwork. I came to "cause of death." I hunched over the paperwork and shielded my face with my hands, to hide the tears that flooded my eyes as I considered the word. "Euthanasia."

Yellow Ooze

Sarah Canavan, MD

HE LIES THERE, without a word. Mr. Torres, a once energetic, silver-haired man who laughed when he admitted to smoking too much, lies motionless in his hospital bed. He is surrounded by humming machines supposedly supporting every need. I am not at all sure they are helping him.

Already he is swollen and bloated, his arms and legs disfigured after weeks of fighting infection. His leaky vessels are too weak to hold the liter after liter of saline forced in, and now the pounds of fluid are simply oozing out of his skin in sticky yellow droplets.

He has not been out of bed in two months. He has tubes in his trachea, stomach, artery, penis, and rectum, and two that end in a large vein just above the entrance to his heart. Every morning at 6:00 he is turned, jostled, tugged, and positioned with a hard X-ray board beneath his back so I can stare at the progress of the fluffy white villain invading his lungs. The infection is eating holes in his lungs, and the bed is eating holes in his heels.

He is bruised, bandaged, cut, blistered, and ulcerated, but his fingertips bother me the most. They preserve an individuality in the midst of an illness that has uprooted him from home and placed him in a standard-issue hospital gown. A plumber, his hands were his livelihood. They hefted metal and cranked wrenches. They also held his daughter's hand as she walked down the aisle. To the right of the ventilator is a picture of him beaming at her wedding, his hands joining her to her husband. Now his hands rest bloated and shiny at his sides, his fingers a bloody pulp, bits of old cotton stuck to the ends. Every hour, a needle punctures his finger, the tip squeezed until it releases a drop of blood, ultimately revealing his blood sugar concentration. There is an order to do this to him, and I have signed it. I can stand in my white coat and speak confidently about the journal article that says we should do this, an article that proves tight blood sugar control improves mortality. But all the pricking and squeezing is absurd, for he is beyond tight blood sugar control. Each morning on rounds when we pass his glass-enclosed room and nod our heads, agreeing that the insulin should be raised just a bit, I silently pray that he not feel the stick inflicted every hour. It seems so unfair to prick a man dying, a man too weak to resist.

In addition to the blood sugar, I am monitoring blood pressure in two locations, heart rate, and breaths per minute. Every day, I recite his sodium and potassium and check the computer to see whether any of the 20 bottles of his blood incubating in the laboratory have grown any new organisms that could be battled with more fluid and antibiotics. I think about him constantly, count his drops of urine, carry ten index cards with tiny black numbers describing him, and know I have been talking about him in my sleep. I know the condition of his organs, a strange and intimate knowledge that gives the illusion of knowing the man behind the numbers.

However, I know only the man reflected in his wife's and daughter's concern and the few pictures that attempt to anchor him beyond this life of tubes, beeping, and pricking. The pictures reveal a man nothing like he is now, too tired to speak, exhausted after turning his head to stare into his wife's eyes.

She shudders when she looks into those blank eyes. It took a week for her to build enough courage to reach his bedside. For the first few days, she was so overwhelmed she could walk only halfway down the hall to his bed, where I would find her clutching the railing, lost in her fear. Now, with stooped shoulders and puffy eyes, she stands beside him. I am amazed at her courage to come into this room and touch his swollen hand, staining her sleeve with the yellow ooze. I don't know how she can enter this room. I can come in only when I force myself and don't look too closely. I hate myself for the helplessness I feel looking at him. I know I shouldn't have such feelings. I am the doctor. I am supposed to do something, anything. I am supposed to be realistic and honest but still impart hope. At the very least, I am supposed to do no harm. I know we are losing, and I fear I am betraying him.

I wish I could say his eyes sparkled when he saw his wife, that there was some recognition of the 45 years and the three children. No. His eyes remain faded, sunken, and focused far beyond the ceiling. It's awful to see him just staring there, his daughter tells me. I nod. What should I do, I wonder, use an extra pillow so he can stare at the wall? I touch her shoulder and she leaves, eyes glistening.

Sometimes I sit with him when I write my notes. I am not sure whether he can hear me, despite the amplifying earphones we have ordered specially for him. Occasionally, he turns his face toward mine. Once, when I was poised above his head, ready to plunge a needle in his neck, I felt him move under the blue sterile drapes covering his face. I lifted the cover to find him shaking his head—no. I reached for the amplifier, dirtying my gloves. Did he understand that he needed this line for the fluids and antibiotics? Or was he asking me to stop the pricking, oozing, and jostling? I summoned his family and watched his wife ask him about the central line. He nodded. She asked again. He nodded again—go ahead. I have never been sure whether perhaps he just couldn't bear to give up in front of his wife, knowing it would hurt her to live without him. I fear I let him down at a time when I could have offered relief and comfort instead of another needle in his neck.

Several days later, his suffering was finally over, new white sheets crisp on his empty bed. That day I thought I saw his wife's shoulders lift just an inch. Why do we know so little about when to let it end? I still talk about him in my sleep.

Transitions

Robert Lamberts, MD

MEDICAL SCHOOL AND residency are times of fear—or at least they were for me. The metamorphosis from college student to doctor kept me up at night with worry. And just prior to moving from the classrooms of the second year in medical school to the hospital wards of the third year, I was especially terrified. All I knew how to do was to study and take tests. If there was a job that required studying and taking tests, I would have been perfectly suited for it. But my internal medicine rotation finally put that anxiety to rest. I wasn't expecting to enjoy it as much as I did, or to excel. The pleasure I had caring for patients and solving problems reassured me that I had, in fact, made the right choice.

Going into residency provoked a different kind of fear. I knew I was capable of the intellectual challenge; it was the physical challenge I feared most. Could I survive call every fourth night and spending most of my waking hours at the hospital? Could I do more than survive it— even enjoy it? Again, the answer was greatly to my relief: I enjoyed it and was even good at it.

So by the time I got to my final year of residency, I was finally in a position of comfort. No matter how acute the problem or how sick the patient, I felt confident in my ability to handle whatever came my way. My training was excellent—I was exposed to a huge number of medical problems, was given ample opportunity to make my own decisions, and was taught by very good clinicians. I was prepared as well as anyone could be prepared. I was ready to move into private practice.

Or so I thought.

I joined another physician, doing both inpatient and outpatient care. Inpatient medicine was a little different for me, but most of the changes were good ones. Calling a surgical consult in residency often resulted in moans, complaints, and even hostility on the other side of the line. In private practice, however, consults are what keep a surgeon in business. They *wanted* me to call!

Seeing a patient with vague abdominal pain one day, I was at the end of my rope. I had done all of the workup I could, and still her pain persisted. Could it be her gallbladder, despite the fact that the ultrasound was negative?

I ordered other tests, tried other treatments, but the pain persisted.

So I called the surgeon. "I have a woman here with abdominal pain. I have done an ultrasound, CT scan, and labs, and have tried her on meds. Nothing has worked. Would you mind taking a look at her for me?"

I prepared for a tongue-lashing. This was not a surgical problem; I had proven that through all of the negative tests. What did I expect the surgeon to do for me? I knew this was the case, but I didn't know what else to do. The response on the other end of the line was unexpected: "Wow. You've done a lot of my work for me. I can't think of what it could be, but I would be delighted to see her for you. Good job—I am not used to having patients so well packaged." *This* was a change I could get used to.

As comfortable and familiar as I was in the hospital, office practice required a huge adjustment on my part. I did have some ambulatory care training in residency, but it was infrequent. Getting to know the patients was extremely difficult if they could see me for only two hours on Wednesday afternoon. Their sicknesses didn't generally happen on this schedule, so I missed out on much of their care. Each visit in the ambulatory clinic was much like the hospital admission—it involved gathering information about everything that happened since I last saw the patient. Any care that was due had to be fit into the visit, as my next encounter with the patient would not be soon.

This mind-set carried over to my private practice. Complicated patients (a staple of internal medicine) would come to the office, and I felt compelled to address every problem at each visit. A routine visit would commonly extend well beyond the allotted time, and the rest of my patients would have to wait. Just when I thought I had addressed every problem, the patient would throw in something else. I was held hostage by any patient with "oh, by the way" questions. How could I ignore something that could be serious?

Once, an elderly man came to the office to establish with me. He had diabetes, hypertension, and chronic low-back pain. He smoked two packs per day. He came with a large bag of medicines from his previous doctor, not sure what each one was for—this was why he was changing doctors. His previous physician had not paid much heed to his diabetes; I had no record of any of the routine monitoring tests I had been taught all diabetics need. But his main concern was a tingling feeling he was getting in his scalp every two weeks or so. He was afraid he was having a stroke.

I was overwhelmed. Not only did I need to sort through his medications and look at his medical records (mostly illegible), but his blood pressure was high, he needed to quit smoking, and I needed to get all of the tests ordered on him. Just the management of his chronic medical problems seemed a daunting task. Add to that the vague symptoms that most concerned him, and I didn't know where to start. Not only did I want to practice good medicine, but I wanted him to trust me as his doctor. How could I do that when I felt so lost?

I did my best to do everything I could for this man—and many more like him. I am sure I overwhelmed them with the myriad of tests and medicine changes I made. And I probably lost patients over this exhaustive practice.

I am not certain when it happened, but eventually I realized that these people were signing up to see me long term. If I didn't handle a problem today, I could just have the patient come back in one or two weeks. Often when I did so, the problem became much less important. I can much more effectively deal with the one or two most important problems and make the patient happy in the process. The added bonus of repeated visits is that I get to know the patient better. Knowing how patients react—whether they overreact or downplay problems—is very helpful in prioritizing treatment.

I don't take sole blame for my attempts to do everything at once. Patients bring their own misconceptions to the table as well. Many people are simply not used to having a long-term relationship with their doctor. They adopt the consumer mentality which values the immediate over the long term. They want their needs to be met as quickly as possible, even though often the best thing is to do nothing but wait and see what happens. This makes many of them look at multiple visits suspiciously—as if they are a mere ploy by the physician to make more money. When I was new in practice, I was especially sensitive to these negative preconceptions from patients. But my job is to do what is best for my patient, and that often means bypass-ing the fast-food mentality of short-term satisfaction and instead working on building a relationship.

I take several approaches to deal with this suspi-cion from the patient, depending on the circumstance. When a person comes in with critically high blood pressure and chest tightness, but is focusing instead on an annoying, itchy rash, I say, "If the house is burning down, you don't cut the lawn." I try not to downplay the annoying nature of the rash, but instead empha-size my concern for the person's care. "I'll take care of the rash once we make sure you aren't having a heart attack."

I've learned to out-advocate patients for their own health needs. When a patient is on my schedule for treat-ment of a sinus infection, and then wants to talk about his diabetes, I have to say, "I need to give that problem the time it deserves. Do you mind if I bring you back next week to talk about that?" Some patients may think I am just trying to increase revenue, but most understand that I am really practicing good medicine.

Having been in practice for over 14 years now, I real-ize that the most important thing I can offer patients isn't medication or good advice; it is me. I can give the best care to people I know—and the better I know them, the better the care. My real job as an internist is not to fix problems or make diagnoses—although these are impor-tant—but instead to walk alongside all my patients as they make the journey of their life.

Some of those journeys I encounter infrequently and with few interventions, in which case my job is to be there if and when something happens. Other journeys are filled with struggle and hardship. My role is to become one of the more important persons in their lives. My job is to do what I can to fix or prevent problems—but also to just be there when they can't be fixed or prevented.

I enjoy fixing problems, figuring out a difficult diagnosis. These things were much of what drew me to internal medicine. I like to solve difficult puzzles, and internal medicine offers many of these. But the fun and excitement now pale in comparison to my satisfaction in the relationships I have built with my patients. My love of medicine can't rest on my ability to fix problems or make diagnoses, because there will be plenty of problems I can't fix and plenty of diagnoses I'll miss. Caring too much about fixing things or diagnosing leads to fear and frustration—something that I felt far more often when I started than I do now.

I still wrestle with the fast-food mentality, especially when people first come to see me. They often seem anxious to get all of the facts in front of me during that first visit, given that the waiting list for new patients is fairly long. They fear that their next visit will be as distant as the first. When I begin to get overwhelmed, I stop and ask them, "What is the most important thing you need me to address today? I want to make sure that does not get lost among the other issues. We will have plenty of time to go after these problems when I see you again." The relief on their face is obvious—as is the surprise.

What does it mean to be an internist? To me, it means that I live through my patients' medical problems with them. I am not the most important person in these relationships; they are. I am the conductor and they are the orchestra. My job is to make sure they are doing everything they can to maximize their health. I put the tools in their hands so they can take care of themselves. Nobody goes to a concert to see the conductor—they want to hear the orchestra. The conductor does the hard work in practice sessions prior to the performance, but the goal is to make the orchestra sound the best it can. I accomplish this over time. I do it by seeing people over and over again.

In a way, my early fear was there because I didn't understand this. I thought that the doctor-patient relationship was limited to my performance, and I was nervous that I would not perform for my patients as I should. Building long-term relationships with people has not only taken the focus off me and so removed my fear, it has removed my patients' fear as well. They know I am there and will be there to help them. If they face difficult times or have medical problems, they know I am there to guide them and work with them.

What better job could there be than removing fear?

Human Contact

Rima Bishara, MD

M R. AND MRS. T are longtime patients of mine. Over time, they have become regular fixtures in the office, coming in for their usual medical care—and sometimes, unusual care.

They are both elderly. She is blind; he has trouble with his joints. They have trouble with their finances, although they are better off than many of their counterparts. They need help to get groceries, because she can't read the product labels and he doesn't know what to buy.

Their last appointment was a micro-view of their lives.

Both came in on the same day because it's cheaper to get someone to drive them at the same time than to come on two separate days. She is concerned about some personal hygiene issues with Mr. T, and he is griping about her cooking.

I listen as they go back and forth. Mrs. T alleges that Mr. T stinks and that he just needs a good bath. He is indignant. She contends that he pees in a can and doesn't wash up. He chimes in that his legs hurt and he can't get to the bathroom overnight, so he uses a can. He insists he empties the can in the morning and that he bathes regularly. Mrs. T used to be a nurse and insists there is something wrong with Mr. T because "he stinks!"

On examination, I note that Mr. T has developed a mild skin infection that needs some treatment and is apparently the cause of his malodorous state. Mr. T says "I told you so!" to Mrs. T, and Mrs. T says "I told you there was something wrong!" right back.

Mrs. T then launches into a diatribe about the fact that Mr. T "won't eat anything I cook for him" and there must be something wrong with his appetite. Mr. T looks at her, then at me, and unleashes his own barrage: "Well, I just don't feel like eating meat all the time. How about some SALAD! We haven't had SALAD in three months. I LOVE SALAD!" He then looks at me and winks, feeling triumphant that he has caught her off guard. She hangs her head and says simply, "Well, okay."

Trying my best to avoid a direct hit while standing between them, I offer some suggestions on getting groceries, and some other community resources they might be able to access to help with this situation.

After spending the remainder of the visit working out social details and revisiting the strategy to help them with their medical and dietary needs, I realize that this was probably the third or fourth time we have worked and reworked the plan. Perhaps the plan is not a good one.

Then, as I am thinking of a major change in approach to include more structured housing (a creative way to say "nursing home"), they both reach out to say thank you in their own way. Mrs. T can't see, but goes on to prattle about this recipe and that and her pastor and the church friends who help them. Mr. T says under his breath, "I'm sure glad we came in today. She's driving me crazy!" They take their time leaving the clinic, talking to each staff member on their way out. They repeat their stories to anyone who will stop and listen. They grab outstretched hands as they walk/wheel their way down the hallway.

Watching them made me think about the role of social contact in cultures where mobility and geographic or societal issues are challenging the nuclear and extended family. Studies about the importance of social interaction in the elderly population are increasing. With the baby boomer generation aging, this will be a critical issue facing us all.

Studies from the United States, Australia, and the United Kingdom all confirm that regular scheduled social contact, even if just once per week, can have an immense impact on the elderly and those who are confined. Some of those studies have even shown that levels of a destructive protein can be lowered by strong social bonds.

People getting regular social contact have reported less loneliness and less social isolation. Social contact also provides a critical link to this group of vulnerable people by allowing a discreet monitoring of their health and welfare. It might be their only link to society at large and the services which might be available to help. These people also reported going to the doctor less often, as well as having a sense of looking forward to something—"a reason to get dressed up."

I realize now that maybe the role I played with Mr. and Mrs. T had nothing to do with medicine, but was really about the social contact I provided. How valuable is this contact to two elderly shut-ins, who look forward to a doctor's office visit as an outlet? Home Health and Meals On Wheels not withstanding, the real value is not in the bandages and pills and food. These things certainly have their value. But, ultimately, it is the human element that soothes the soul and quiets the nerves.

If that happens to be at the doctor's office, well, why not?

Tiffany

Lee Savio Beers, MD

Tiffany was 15 years old when I first met her, with her newborn daughter. I noticed that her diaper bag had about ten laminated cards hanging from the shoulder strap. "What are these?" I asked. A little embarrassed, she replied, "I took a parenting class while I was pregnant, and I made them there. They gave me the diaper bag, too." She showed me what was written on the cards—each one had a handwritten sentence describing something positive about herself. I don't remember exactly what they said, but they described a strong, loving young woman. "In the class, they said we could carry these around and look at them every day to help us remember that we can be good parents."

Three years later, I can still see the young woman described in those simple, affirming statements. I don't know if it was the cards, but despite many very serious and ongoing challenges, I think Tiffany, now an adult, is the parent she hoped she would be.

Tiffany had not had an easy childhood. Born into an impoverished, single-parent family in Washington, D.C., she has suffered from many of the problems that accompany extreme poverty. Worse, her own mother frequently sabotages her efforts to make things better for herself and her young daughter. For example, when Tiffany began seeking regular medical care in our clinic, her mother re-enrolled all her children in Medicaid except for her, and then for months refused to sign the paperwork to get her enrolled. Her mother takes many of the benefits intended for Tiffany for herself, leaving Tiffany to scrounge for money to buy things as basic as food and diapers.

When I first met Tiffany, she was sleeping at home on a couch with her newborn, in a room with multiple holes and leaks in the ceiling in an apartment with rats in the kitchen. She tried to have herself removed from her mother's custody so that she could enroll in school near her aunt in Maryland, where she had found a more comfortable and stable home. After many unanswered phone calls, she waited all day in the offices of Child Protective Services, refusing to leave until someone would come out and talk to her; she was ultimately told that there was no justification for removing her from her family's care and that (at least this was her understanding of the situation) if she did not start attending school back in D.C., necessitating a move back in with her mother, she would risk having her own daughter taken away.

She wanted to go to college and be a social worker, so she set her sights on graduating from high school. Since I have known her, she has been in five schools. One school was too far away from her child's day care, and she was always an hour late. Another never gained accreditation, leaving her no credits for a year spent in classes. Her mother wouldn't sign the paperwork to send her back to a residential school, where she was thriving academically despite some struggles with the very regimented structure. Now she is enrolled in a GED program, just ten credits away from graduation. "I just can't wait any longer," she told me. Every time I see her, I hear about some new and serious challenge she has faced. Yet she keeps moving forward, dealing with each new obstacle. No matter what is happening, she continues to come see me and the staff in my clinic who have gotten to know her well, more for the social support and encouragement, I think, than for the medical care. We do all that we can to help her, but unfortunately there are limits to what we can do in a city with broken schools and inadequate access to a host of other services.

I wish I could know where she will ultimately end up. While she is legally an adult now, she is still an adolescent, developing her sense of self and making her own way in the world. She has so much in front of her, and also so much behind her. I hope that she keeps fighting because I see all her potential. I think she sees it too, and that is why she hasn't given up. What I do know is that she is a patient and loving parent. She is often reading to her daughter when I enter the exam room. She distracts or redirects her when she begins to act out, instead of yelling. Her family tells her she should "beat" her daughter to "get her to behave," but she tells me very emphatically, "I am not going to hit my child." Indeed, her daughter is a lovely, charming, and cheerful little girl—certainly, she has her moments, but then so does my own three-year-old.

I hope some day to hear about Tiffany's wonderful accomplishments, and that she and her family are living in a warm and stable environment. As we know from the life story of President Obama, who is himself the son of a teenage mother, no dream is too great. Most importantly, I want to see her happy with what her life, and her daughter's life, has become; my ideas of success may not ultimately be hers, but that is okay.

For the past five years, I have been the director of a clinic for teen parents, and one important thing I have learned is that Tiffany's story is not as unusual as most think. The horrible things many of these young mothers and fathers face would seem insurmountable to me in my life today, much less when I was a teenager, when I was lucky enough to have a devoted and supportive family. Even more important is the fact that so many of the young parents I care for show the same resilience and desire to change things for their own children that I see in Tiffany.

Of course, there are patients who aren't able to cope with their own life experiences, addictions, or mental health issues. I will always remember the young mother who told me that, yes, her one-year-old was saying her first words . . . b**** and f***. Our program has had patients who were raped, shot, kidnapped, beaten, and even murdered. The rates of violence exposure are astonishingly high, even in a city known for its violence. My staff and I regularly have to struggle to decide where poverty ends and neglect begins. We have to recognize that sometimes we can change a life with a simple action, and sometimes we make little difference despite heroic efforts. Some days I arrive home inspired by something a patient has accomplished, and some days I arrive home drained and a little burned out. I feel as though I have seen and heard it all, even in the relatively short time I have worked with teen parents, but I know, sadly, I really haven't.

Many of my colleagues are very glad that they do not have my job—we don't mind seeing teen parents, they tell me, because we can send them to you. It seems to work out because I love to see them. It makes me smile when a young mother pokes her head into my office just to say hi, or I see a teen father playing peek-a-boo with his new baby. I love seeing the potential in these young parents and enjoy watching it blossom. When someone has very few resources, as many of my patients do, it gives you a chance to see what things are really important. You don't need a house full of toys, a new car, or elaborate vacations to have a loving, thriving, family. Really, all you need is a stack of cards reminding you of all you can do with your love, patience, and determination.

My Calling

Conrad Fischer, MD

I AM AN INFECTIOUS diseases doctor. I have been taking care of HIV-positive patients for 20 years. When I first heard of HIV, I was 19 years old, a college student working as a teaching assistant for a physiology professor in 1982. The professor was an enormous character, a classroom performer with oddball mannerisms and completely unfunny jokes that he told with such good humor that we laughed just to make him happy and because it made us feel good.

"They say it will achieve bubonic plague proportions," he called out from the other room.

"What will?" I asked, confused.

"AIDS," he said. "I just got back from a meeting. It's all they are talking about."

I was typing up his class notes and doing research with electron microscopy on thyroid glands for a reason I cannot possibly remember now, but I knew I had to go to medical school. It became my driving passion. Looking back, I now understand what the word *calling* means: that for reasons you cannot name, you simply MUST do something. As a self-centered, not very compassionate teenager, I decided at the age of 18 that I had to go to medical school at any cost. I had been in a hospital on only the rarest occasions. No one in my family was sick. No one I knew had an incurable disease that I felt driven to cure or treat.

My major concerns were getting the grades I needed to get into medical school and finishing college within three years, because I knew everything else would be long. But the main reason was that I was in a hurry, in a mad rush to become a doctor. I could not have told you why, really. I wanted to change the world, to make a difference. And phrases like that were the ones I rehearsed in a mirror while preparing for medical school interviews. It would take at least another ten years before I stumbled on the reason for my calling: the nameless impulse to do some good in the world, to leave it better than I found it.

* * *

How do you know whether your career choice is right? I am often asked this by medical students struggling to choose a specialty. The answer for me is always, "If you did not have to work for a living, what would you choose to do?" Answer that, and then you will know your choice is right.

I had such a moment one day in the emergency department, seeing patients and teaching. The resident commented, "Wow, Dr. Fischer, you're a really smart guy . . . You should go on one of those TV game shows and win a million dollars."

I thought about this and said, "You know what I would do if I did that and won a million dollars? I would be here with you, right now, doing exactly what we are doing." My answer helped me to realize that I really am living in my calling, although as a 19-year-old applicant to medical school I could not have explained it to you.

Over the years, I have learned that in order to best understand the treatment of HIV as my calling, it is important to hear about the lives of the patients themselves. Their stories have become part of mine. Many of my patients have been very happy to tell their stories, to share their struggles. However, there is a vast difference in how willing they are to have their names attached to their stories. Two are clearly out in the open about their status. Another uses only a nickname, known to a few family members who know her status. Another was so anxious that she was worried even to have her initials used.

* * *

Despite advances in treatment, the social stigma of HIV remains considerable because of the disease's methods of transmission: sexual contact and needle-sharing drug use.

I must point out that several of these patients are hetero-sexual women who would never have found out their status if testing was done only according to risk factors. The implications of this should be enormous: you simply cannot tell for sure who is HIV-positive by "looking at them."

"I believe in family. The most frightening thing for me was thinking I would not be there for my children. I feel fortunate, and blessed, very blessed to have two healthy children while being HIV-positive."

Li, 42 years old, HIV-positive for 12 years

Li is the mother of two small children. Twelve years ago, she began to feel short of breath. Her doctors told her she had asthma and treated her with inhalers, which did not work. Over several months, she progressed to the point of being in a coma, losing 50 pounds, and being placed in an intensive care unit for pneumonia. On an HIV test, she tested positive. Her husband at the time was unable to understand or accept what was going on. He was HIV-negative, and the transmission was from a boyfriend in the past who she now thinks knew his positive status at the time but did not tell her.

Her husband left her. She recalls, "I was a hundred pounds and could not get out of bed for months. I was weak and fragile and could not take care of myself. My rent went unpaid and the bills were piling up. He left me just when I needed him the most." Li made a slow recovery and was fortunate to have found out her HIV status in 1996, when it had just become clear that combination antiretroviral therapy was highly effective. She continued to improve and is now somewhat overweight and much happier.

"Be careful who you tell," she cautioned. "I lost a lot of friends at the time who could not accept it. My parents found out and they were my main support, but they are old-timers and they thought I was going to die at any moment. I believe in family. I was pregnant with my son, and all I thought about was having a healthy baby," she told me.

Li was severely anemic at the time I met her, during her first pregnancy. Because of this, she could not take AZT, the original medication that prevents the mother-to-child transmission of HIV, because that medication can cause anemia. She also would not take a blood transfusion because of her own personal beliefs rooted in, I believe, an upbringing as a Jehovah's Witness. Because of the other HIV medications, and luck, her child today is healthy and beautiful. Li's HIV, although resistant to multiple medications, is sufficiently controlled to allow her to lead a normal life—at least physically.

"I thank God for the medications. Also, if you are HIV-positive and they ask you to volunteer for research on new medications, you should do it." When I asked her whether she feels fortunate, Li replied, "There is always someone worse off than you. Cancer will eat you up alive in no time. I had a cousin who got bitten by a mosquito and died of dengue a few weeks later, and left three small children with no mother."

*"Please don't even use my initials. I am scared
someone will know I'm HIV-positive."*

Anonymous, 48, HIV-positive for 14 years
"Anonymous" found out in 1989 that she was HIV-positive
when she went to donate blood for her sick child. She was
the only person I interviewed who would not allow the
use of her name or even her initials. In the age of reality
TV, everyone wants to tell their story. And while Anonymous is no different in terms of her desire to be known,
you have to understand the kind of fear that goes along
with HIV. I choose to use this name rather than making
up a false one, because the word *anonymous* reminds us
of how isolating having HIV can be and how far our society still has to go in terms of accepting people with this
illness.

"When my son was sick," she told me, "he needed
surgery on an aneurysm. I was stunned to find I was
positive. I wasn't promiscuous. I wasn't a drug user. My
husband was HIV-negative. The only thing I can think
of was a blood transfusion I had received several years
before. All I thought about was 'please, God, let me live
long enough to take care of my son.' I did not realize
what this meant for myself until later. I never expected
to live this long."

"How were you told?" I asked.

"They called up over the phone and told me. All I
remember was they told me never to have any more kids,"
she said.

HIV has a tremendous effect on families, but not always in the way Li described previously. Anonymous said, "My husband became consumed with my being HIV-positive. All he did was research to try and find a way to help me. He was driving me crazy really. Finally, I had to leave him. I felt I was holding him back. I felt he should be with someone like him who was healthy. He couldn't understand. He is still my best friend. To this day, he still calls me up and says, 'You know what, I just heard about this new treatment.' I know HIV had a lot to do with us breaking up."

When I asked her what she is grateful for, she acknowledged the medications that keep her alive and the tolerance that HIV has taught her. These days, she has a new and great relationship with a man who is also HIV-positive, whom she met through an online dating service for HIV-positive people.

Apparently, the tolerance that Anonymous feels for others is not always reciprocated by others. Hence, the compulsion to completely hide her identity.

Are we, as a profession, tolerant? Are we tolerant of behavior issues related to sex and drug use, and do we use a "disease model," the only one proven effective to help people?

When we think of the importance of medical research, do we also think about the intense need to move fast? Do we consider that when one person is ill, it is never just one person, but the whole group of people around that person? For example, when my own sister-in-law died of

AIDS, just a few months short of living long enough for newly developed protease inhibitors to snatch her from the jaws of death, my brother died with her, quite possibly of a broken heart.

"It was only when I met my doctor that I did not wake up every day thinking I was going to die."

Billy Fields, 57, HIV-positive for 16 years

Billy Fields is a completely out-in-the-open gay, HIV-positive man. I have been his doctor for 14 years. He can tell me the exact day that he found he was HIV-positive, because it was the same day his father died. Billy has a new type of faith in his caregiver; although he implicitly trusts me, he *always* does enormous homework.

"You have to educate yourself. You can't go in to the doctor and just say 'I am sick.' You have to look into things. In this type of environment," he told me, "you have to work harder than your doctor. You have more time than they do, so go to the library or the Internet and find out about things. Then be selective in who you choose as a doctor. Make sure it is someone you can talk to and stick with him. But make sure you come into the visit with information."

I asked Billy whether he ever saw this as contradictory for the doctor-patient relationship. On the contrary, he has tremendous faith in me personally not to let him down. However, he never just sits back and lets me tell him what to do. This is a phenomenon that really developed with the advent of HIV infection but has become more widespread. Your doctor is now, in a way, your consultant in your own investigations and choices. Some doctors do not like this. They feel that the patients are too pushy and independent. But Billy shows us that an independent-minded, well-educated patient who already knows a lot of medicine is every bit as grateful as a passive one. The sense of kinship is not less—if anything, it seems to be more.

Also, for my own part, I realized that this decreases my burden as a physician. If the patient is passive, never learns anything, and just follows commandments, then any error is 100 percent my fault. I did not realize this until speaking to Billy. Partnership with an educated patient does not inhibit the growth of the real human relationship that is the heart of our profession.

I asked Billy what frightens him most about the disease. He responded, "When I get sick and I do not know what will happen. I also feel like I let you down when I get sick." I had never heard something like this from a patient before.

I also asked Billy whether he lost any relationships when he became positive. "Oh no! My family is very supportive. And if you were going to lose friends, then it is better to find out right away, because they weren't really your friend to begin with. My mother always told us, 'When someone gets sick, come calling!' so in my family and with my friends I only got closer to people. I have tremendous friends who go way out of their way to help me. And I go take care of other people when they get sick."

When we talked about his motivation to go on, I was both stunned and amused by the response: "I love to play tennis! I want to stay alive to play tennis!" Also, he says, "You have to be involved, to do something to make sure funding is there. You have to play your part. It is kind of like a child saying, 'What did you do in the war, Daddy?'—you have to do something. That is why I sit on committees and go to the capital to lobby for money for treatment."

So as long as they are engaged with life, no matter what that engagement is, people have a reason to live.

> *"Having access to the medications is like*
> *carrying around a million-dollar check."*
>
> Martina Clark, 44, HIV-positive for 16 years

After many years of seeing the same patients, I recently started taking new ones. I went into the waiting area, and as I scanned the room, I noticed someone very atypical. I thought, "Who is the well-dressed, attractive lady with the blue eyes, blond hair, and stylish scarf? It must be an administrator or a drug company representative." I quickly moved on and called out for my next patient. "Martina Clark?"

To my surprise, the stylish lady stood up and walked over. Twenty years after graduating from medical school, I had an eye-contact "moment" with a patient for the first time. "This is weird," I thought. By the time I got back in the exam room, however, I had reestablished my professionalism.

Martina was my age, 44, at the time. She was an educated, extremely well-traveled heterosexual white woman with no risk factors for HIV. She has known she was positive since 1992 when, living in San Francisco, she had the fever, fatigue, and rash we now know is associated with acute infection with HIV. Her story was a compelling one: "They did not know what I had. I did not fit. But, seeing as I was a single woman in San Francisco and not knowing what else to do, they tested me for HIV. They gave me my diagnosis over the phone . . . They didn't know what to do with me, but told me I would most likely be dead within five years. There wasn't much available in terms of medications at that time, and my T cells were still high, so I was not on therapy. I did not know what to do, so I went to a support group. I hated it. It seemed like a lot of people sitting around complaining and feeling sorry for themselves.

"I decided to take a different route and became, for lack of a better word, an activist. I figured if I was going to die soon, I wanted to make sure that my life had some meaning and that I did something with it. Overnight, I developed 'AIDS star syndrome.' I went to the White House; I met Bill Clinton. I got recruited by the United Nations AIDS program, and I now work with the HIV in the Workplace program worldwide. I knew that I had to do something. I knew that I was atypical. As an educated white woman, I knew I had more access to have my voice heard than others, so I had to fight back. This is what gave my life purpose and at least, at that time, gave me energy. I am grateful that there are medications, even though I have not had to use them, because it is like walking around with a million-dollar check in your pocket. I have been in 78 countries. But now I just want to be normal."

Martina was extremely lucid and clear. Drug development really is promising. And she was grateful for a lot of things, but the social stigma of HIV and the profound loneliness that can come with it are still heartbreaking. She intimated that she still feels simultaneously the pain of isolation and the good fortune of access to care. "It's not like I am a woman in rural Malawi. I know if I get sick, there are options." But she added, "At this point, I would just be happy to have a boyfriend, sing in a band, and do some pottery."

* * *

I recently thought about whether I was sure I had ever saved someone's life. It is hard to be sure. People we resuscitate often slip back and die anyway. The greatest number of lives I have ever saved, for sure, was not done with a prescription, a procedure, or a device. The greatest number of lives I have ever saved was from working to pass pediatric AIDS legislation, which has led to the virtual elimination of children with AIDS in the United States. The greatest success—in terms of number of lives—has been from fighting and from using *all* my voices. Not from forcing my head and my mannerisms into a vise so that people would accept me, although I certainly tried to do this, but rather from finding the precise part of the world that needed my abilities. Liabilities in one area, when moved somewhere else, are often called talents.

These are the same qualities that have made me a pain in the ass to authority figures. The same qualities that made me too large, loud, and clumsy to get into a lab made me just right to fight back and win this war, for Billy, Li, Anonymous, and Martina.

THE DOCTOR'S WIFE

Sayantani DasGupta, MD, MPH

MY HUSBAND BRINGS his work home. Had he been a butcher, it might have been a prime cut of steak; a mason, a block of limestone. The newspaper reporter brings home fingers covered in ink; and the fishmonger, the smell of the sea. But my husband is an oncologist, so he brings home the dead and dying.

This makes our king-size bed rather crowded. The children, padding into the room after midnight on footie-pajamaed feet to cuddle beside us, are unaware of who is already there between their parents: a bald 33-year-old woman who will never be a mother, a grieving widow who turned her anger against her husband's doctor rather than his horrible disease, a beloved grandfather whose cancer has metastasized to every far-reaching corner of his body. My husband's patients hog the blankets, steal my pillow, shake the mattress with their sobs.

Over the sleeping body of our curly-haired daughter, my husband and I watch the television pundits discuss the war in Iraq, then a human-interest story about the young men and women, not really that much older than our own babies, who carry guns, drive tanks, and watch their comrades suffer and die. We stare at the screen in silence, together and apart, fixed on images of young bodies killing and being killed.

Even on returning home, some soldiers can never be the same. Violent memories linger, recurring like tumors. After so much blood, some soldiers become dry and still like stones.

"The only difference," my husband finally says, "is that those soldiers see death like a flash—quick and fierce and chaotic." With his index finger, he gently traces the baby's slightly parted lips—a perfect cupid's bow. Then he looks away. "I watch people die in slow motion."

In medical school, they called us marines. Osler marines, to be precise, after the venerable Dr. William, who, so they say, was a general of a man. We were in the trenches, on the front lines, soldiering on. Antibiotics bombed infections, diligent docs were gunners, and incoming patients were middle-of-the-night hits to be avoided.

It was no time to be at war with metaphor. Metaphor was at war with us and winning by a big margin.

In our white-coated uniforms, our scrub-suit camouflage, we were the measly privates of the operation being taught the ways of battle. We were given rounds of bullets with names like distance, objectivity, and self-preservation. Any other kind of medical practice was strictly on a don't-ask, don't-tell basis.

So we huddled together for warmth in the foxholes of training. In the field, almost a dozen couples were born—all fair in love and war—among them, my husband and me.

"Medicine makes a jealous mistress," our teachers told us laughingly, even as our dean earnestly recommended that I reconsider obstetrics for pediatrics, a field more suited to family life and what is, after all, a military marriage.

What is it to witness continuous suffering? What is it to continuously witness suffering? Emmanuel Levinas posited that the ethical work of medicine lies in this act of witnessing—of seeing the Other's *face*, answering the call of another's suffering.[1] But what philosopher can account for the *weight* of suffering—not only upon those who suffer, but upon those who stand beside suffering? What is the cost of ethical practice? What is the responsibility of those who witness the experience of witnesses?

Historically, medicine recognized the need for physicians to be witnessed, even as they were witnessing their patients. In part, this need was satisfied by the Hegelian sense of recognition, whereby the gift of recognition was returned: patients could engage with and recognize the humanity of their doctor, who in turn engaged with and recognized theirs.[2] This sort of medicine provided other avenues for recognition as well, in local communities in which physicians lived, practiced, and enjoyed special status, and in families in which (male) physicians' (female) partners provided unconditional love and support.

The increasing impersonalization of medicine takes a toll on the ability of physicians to practice ethical medicine—medicine in which they not only diagnose but *see* their patients. This is due not only to shortened visit times, increased patient loads, and a reliance on technological data over interpersonal interaction, but to a disintegration of avenues whereby physicians are themselves *seen*. The loss of support communities around the witnesses to suffering and the lack of social or professional recognition of the toll on witnessing leaves the burden upon relatively isolated spouses. And doctor's wives aren't all what they used to be.

My husband is not yet 40, but he is bowed over like an old man from all the bodies on his back. He carries his patients' stories with him like comrades who have fallen in the field, unable to put them to rest. He mulls and worries about even the ones who make it, cherishing their cards and gifts the way I cherish our children's finger paintings, their construction-paper artwork.

"You're like the son we never had, doctor," I overheard an elderly patient say to him one day, beaming and patting him on the cheek. *Like I don't have enough demanding in-laws*, I thought.

Perhaps I wouldn't be so resentful if it were at least sufficient. But even such a loving gesture cannot outweigh the burden of so many patients, so much suffering and loss. Or perhaps it *could* be enough if he had a moment to sit with her and let her generosity wash over him. But the charts pile up on his door—of the patient with a deforming tumor, the one with interminable questions from the Internet, the one drowning in sorrow and confusion.

Or is the problem that I am a doctor too and can't muster a sufficient sense of awe about my husband's work? The realization lies heavy in my stomach.

"I saw him first," I want to tell them all.

It is a holy practice—or so my friend, another doctor's wife, likes to say, especially those nights her husband doesn't come back until long after she has gone to bed. "It is God's work," she tells me firmly, when my voice trembles from frustration; when I ask questions about *when* and *why* and *is it fair.* She is a banker and hates her job. She swallows her spouse's sorrows with her own.

I tell her the story of Psyche, who was forbidden to look upon her beloved, Cupid—whose only encounters with him were in the dark. One night, tormented by the need to *see,* she held aloft an oil lamp and illuminated his sleeping form. She was so overcome by the beauty of his face that she spilled hot oil on his shoulder. Startled awake and realizing her betrayal, her injured husband stretched his wings and flew away, leaving her quite alone.

"Peek-a-boo," my friend says, to no one in particular.

After the news program, I decide to read aloud Raymond Carver's poem "The Autopsy Room." I read it instead of stroking my husband's hair, or asking him to tell me—*please* tell me. I have tried these tacks. Our daughter still slumbers between us, mewing and twitching—I cannot guess what she's dreaming about either.

I read the poem because it's about a husband who has witnessed too much and a wife who tries to understand. The young man is not a doctor, but cleans a morgue where bodies and body parts are at times left on the coroner's table. Among them:

> A *little baby,*
> *still as stone and snow cold,* . . .
> *a huge black man with white hair whose chest*
> *had been laid open,* . . .
> *a pale and shapely leg.*[3]

My husband listens, silent and immobile. For a moment, I wonder if he is sleeping with his eyes open.

Once home, Carver's narrator is paralyzed—quaking like those first anatomists—because he has been to the forbidden temple, he has entered the Medusa's cave, he has *seen.* He stares at the ceiling, the floor. But then his wife takes his hand to her breast, saying,

> "Sugar, it's going to be all right. We'll trade
> in this life for another."[4]

His fingers stray to her leg, which is alive, warm, and willing. But he remains in limbo between this world and the next, unable to return to the shores of the living.

"I'm Charon the ferryman," my husband finally says, breaking his silence. "I'm a shaman to the spirit-world."

Our daughter turns over in her sleep, fitful.

With my words and images, I will weave a yellow ribbon of remembrance and tie it around our bedpost—a beacon home for my beloved.

. . . *Nothing*
was happening. Everything was happening.[5]

I see you, I try to say, but my voice trips and stumbles.

. . . *Life*
was a stone, grinding and sharpening.[6]

NOTES

[1] C. Irvine, "The Other Side of Silence: Levinas, Medicine, and Literature," *Literature & Medicine* 24, no. 1 (2005): 8–18.

[2] J. Butler, *Giving an Account of Oneself* (New York: Fordham University Press, 2005).

[3] R. Carver, "The Autopsy Room," in *On Doctoring: Stories, Poems, Essays,* ed. R. Reynolds and J. Stone (New York: Simon & Schuster, 1991), 367–68.

[4] Ibid.

[5] Ibid.

[6] Ibid.

INDISCRETIONS

Anna Reisman, MD

YOU HEAR ABOUT the biggies: the ones that make the papers, the ones that have the hospital staff buzzing. The ones that might end up being analyzed by quality management teams or during a morbidity and mortality conference: a megadose of potassium killing a patient, a wrong leg amputated, a lung mass missed on an X-ray.

Few, if any, hear about the near misses and close calls. The uncomfortable reality, though, is that the little mistakes occur far more frequently than anyone would care to admit. And while most of us keep them to ourselves and may eventually forget them, it's plain that we can learn as much from the little ones as we can from the whoppers.

Here is a little one of my own.

I was returning calls for a colleague who was out of town. A Mrs. Dessaint answered the phone. In a soft Southern drawl, she told me that her husband had asked her to call in for his cholesterol result.

As medical students, we're taught that without specific permission from the patient, we shouldn't give out results to anyone else. But many of us do it anyway, particularly if the results are normal. For whatever reason—our patient load is overwhelming, we're backed up on charts—we just don't have time to keep calling.

And that was one of those days. It was late; it was raining; I was rushing to make a train. Cradling the phone between my left shoulder and ear, standing over my desk with my coat on, I found the chart among the five or six that remained on my desk and opened it to the lab section. Mr. Dessaint was young, just 34, so I didn't expect any surprises. Normal. Normal. Normal. "Looks pretty good," I heard myself saying into the receiver, "normal cholesterol, normal blood sugar." I flipped to the previous page. And stared.

Gonorrhea culture: positive.

An uneasiness washed through me. I lowered myself into my chair. I told Mrs. Dessaint that one test had come back abnormal, but I couldn't give out any further information; her husband needed to call back himself. From the way she paused, I could tell she suspected it was something bad. How could she not? Her voice creased with concern, she told me her husband was working the late shift and wouldn't be home until 11:00.

Was it better to leave her imagining the worst—and I was sure she was thinking cancer or HIV—or just tell her the truth? It was unlikely that waiting the few days until Mr. Dessaint called back would lead to any adverse health effects. Still, I couldn't help myself from picturing a double-screen image: on one side, a delicate Mrs. Dessaint in the emergency room, shaking with chills, blood leaking from her vagina, a festering abscess growing on her fallopian tubes; on the other, her swaggering husband stopping off at a local strip joint to talk up some tart with double-D breast implants. *She deserves to know,* I thought. *It's curable. She should be tested right away. In the end, she'll be grateful.*

The words spilled out. She gasped. I heard the phone clatter to the ground. I told Mrs. Dessaint what she needed to do and hung up. Heart pounding, I grabbed my bag, dashed through the gray drizzle to my car, and sped to the station. I made the train just as the doors slammed shut.

In retrospect, my lapse of judgment seemed stunning. This was privileged information. Absent explicit permission from the patient, I would never tell a patient's husband that her mammogram showed a suspicious mass. I would never give someone other than the patient an HIV test result. What I had done was extraordinarily presumptuous: not taking a moment to consider how upsetting it might be to hear—from a doctor, no less—that your husband had a sexually transmitted disease with promiscuity written all over it.

At the same time, gonorrhea was a reportable disease, and it was indisputably my duty to inform. Of course, it was not my duty to inform the patient's wife. That was Mr. Dessaint's decision, not mine. Had I waited until I was able to reach him and asked him to come to the office, I could have urged him to disclose his diagnosis to his wife. If he refused, I could have pointed out that I had to report it to the local department of health and she would find out anyway. In retrospect, how simple it might have been!

This kind of back-and-forth went on all weekend. I wanted to protect her, to ensure that she would be okay. But what I had done was wrong; it flew in the face of one of the most basic tenets of medicine, patient confidentiality. And my reasons were simply that it was gray and raining and I wanted to get out of the clinic and make my train. But maybe there were deeper reasons as well. Had I let my visceral hostility to Mr. Dessaint's behavior take over for what were likely his gross indiscretions?

Back in my clinic on Monday, I pulled Mr. Dessaint's chart. There were considerable grounds for me to be sued, and I needed to document my reasoning; perhaps someone on the jury would understand that I had been attempting to do the right thing. I opened the chart to the telltale page. And froze. The gonorrhea test was from a year earlier. A barely legible note indicated that he had been treated. This was old news.

Hands shaking, I dialed Mrs. Dessaint. A deep male voice on the other end sharply told me that no one by that name lived there. I said that I was a doctor, which got someone else on the phone, who said she was at work. I called again after lunch and spoke with her grandmother, who repeated she didn't live there and didn't know what her phone number was. Two days later I had gotten nowhere. Maybe it was already too late—maybe she had already left her husband, or shot him, or castrated him. Finally, on Friday, I pleaded with her grandmother to pass along the message that I was terribly sorry, I had been mistaken about some results I gave to Mrs. Dessaint, she shouldn't worry. I left the grandmother both my office and home numbers.

At times that week, I found myself wondering whether I could blame my oversight on the system, argue that the lab or the medical records department had mixed up the page with the gonorrhea result and the current labs. But in the end my better judgment told me to be honest. I was ready to come clean, if only I could reach the Dessaints.

Then, on Saturday night, the phone rang. "She's not here," I snapped to the unfamiliar female voice, presuming a telemarketer, but suddenly I recognized the mellow lilt. Mrs. Dessaint. She got her husband on another phone. After yammering on for what seemed like a long time, I took a breath. There was silence on the other end of the line. I started over. "I misread a report," I said, "and I'm so sorry that I worried you." I cringed, expecting an angry reaction. To my surprise, they had little to say. They thanked me before hanging up.

Seven years later, I haven't been slapped with a complaint from the Dessaints. Perhaps this is because I admitted my error promptly and took responsibility for it; studies have shown that frank disclosure of mistakes not only reduces lawsuits but improves the doctor-patient relationship. Or perhaps it can be explained by the fact that there was no bad outcome. But sometimes I find myself wondering if what I did in some small way punctured the bond of trust between a husband and wife and introduced a leak into their relationship that could, or did, sink their marriage. There's no way to measure such subtle effects of a mistake, of course. I can only hope my indiscretion faded from the Dessaints' memory as the years wore on and that it was eventually forgotten. But I won't forget it. For me, it was a biggie.

ON CARING FOR DIFFICULT PATIENTS

Tony Miksanek, MD

L ET'S BE BLUNT. It's hard to care for difficult patients. It's sometimes impossible to actually like them. This species of sick individuals tends to strain time, patience, and resources. They often generate a cascade of phone calls. They sometimes demand a heap of medically unnecessary tests. They occasionally refuse recommended treatment. Many have unreasonable expectations. Some whine and gripe incessantly. A few threaten to sue. Almost all of them need at least 30 minutes—and want 60 minutes—of face time with the doctor at every encounter instead of the usual 15 minutes the schedule actually allows.

In more than 20 years of general practice in a very small town, I can claim only a tiny number of demanding patients who have made my life difficult—much less than 1 percent. Consider three patients all seen by me in the same week. In their own unique ways, they make my professional life tricky. Even in my private life, they invade my thoughts—with disappointment, irritation, and worry.

Willy is a great guy, even though he's a lousy patient. The 37-year-old salesman was diagnosed with type 1 diabetes 14 years ago. He has been my patient for three years. I treat his father and mother; they asked me to accept their son as a patient. They said that he was looking for a "good doctor." Little did I know that "good doctor" meant any physician unfamiliar with his history and naïve enough to take him as a patient.

It turns out that Willy had burned his bridges with most of the other local physicians. He didn't have many doctors left to choose from in our rural area; I might have been the only name left on the list. At his first office visit, he made his intentions quite clear.

"Look, Doc, I'm not going to waste your time. All I need is a prescription for my insulin and syringes. I'm a decent patient. I'll never bother you."

What doctor wouldn't be enamored by the promise of never being bothered? I never thought such a thing was possible.

After a thorough history and physical examination during that initial visit, the man had me convinced of his benign nature. His blood pressure was excellent. Pulses were strong. His feet were in good condition. There was no sign of any damage to his eyes from diabetes.

I began blabbering about diabetic care. I gave him a laundry list of lab tests to get done and insisted he call or fax one week's worth of his blood sugar values—taken at least twice a day—to the office for my review. Willy was courteous and listened intently up to that point, but he couldn't take any more.

"Whoa!" he interrupted me. "I've got it covered. No problem. All I need are some refills."

Willy apprised me that he managed his blood sugars and adjusted the insulin dose on his own. He wasn't asking for my assistance. He confessed he had no sliding-scale system or arithmetical formula to guide his insulin management; instead he relied on intuition and personal experience.

"No offense to you, Doc," Willy apologized. "I know my body pretty well. I've got a good track record in 14 years—no passing out from low blood sugars; no being put in the hospital because my sugar was way too high."

And then he flashed a smile and patted me on the back. It was role reversal. His gesture was supposed to make everything all right—his need for absolute autonomy, his uncanny ability to control a serious disease, and my relegation to a pen and prescription pad. At that moment all I could think was, "Damn, this guy's a good salesman."

What self-respecting physician would relinquish total control of a complex illness to a patient? None that I know.

That answer was corroborated by the later knowledge that Willy had been "fired" by a few doctors in the area. I suggested a referral to an endocrinologist. There are only two of them within 90 miles of our town. Willy refused without offering any reason, even though he might have offered distance as an excuse. He also made it clear that he would come to the office only once a year. It was his way or no way.

I had a choice to make. If I refused to treat Willy, where else could he go? Perhaps I could change his behavior. Maybe I could succeed where my peers had failed. Willy was polite and funny and hardworking and smart. Most important, he seemed incapable of lying. He believed that he knew his body better than any doctor. He never alleged that he understood the physiology of diabetes and the intricacies of insulin.

His glycohemoglobin A1c (a blood test that measures the average sugar for the past two to three months) at that first office visit was 7.5 percent—not ideal, but not too bad for a do-it-yourselfer (a normal value is less than 6 percent). I wrote him refill prescriptions for needles and syringes along with two types of insulin: NPH (an intermediate-acting form that he injects twice a day) and Regular (a short-acting form). He refused to consider changing his insulin to Lantus, a newer, long-acting one that he would need to inject only once a day. He promised that he would continue regularly monitoring his blood sugars at home. I shuddered to think what he considered "regularly."

True to his word, Willy never bothers me. He faithfully comes to my office once a year but never more. At this week's visit, I wrote refill prescriptions for him. I worry about Willy, but what can I do? If I cut him loose, how will he fend for himself? Will he find a friendly pharmacist to do his bidding? Or purchase insulin over the Internet?

At the conclusion of this week's appointment with Willy, I performed a little self-analysis. Why do I picture him as a difficult patient? Obviously, he isn't playing by the rules—at least not the rules I learned in medical school. He won't allow me to do my job. If I can't control his treatment, I'd at least appreciate a 50 percent stake in it. I aim for perfection. Willy's goal is just getting along with his disease on friendly terms and avoiding hassles or complications. If his chart is ever reviewed by the insurance company for quality of care, I'm going to get dinged. At the same time, Willy's self-reliance might offer a lesson about controlling health care costs and empowering patients. Still, I need to quit coddling Willy. What makes me an ineffective physician in my mind is exactly the quality that Willy deems vital in his primary care doctor: I'm easy.

* * *

In contrast to Willy, I can never do enough for Mrs. Thomasina. The 81-year-old widow is in good health except for high blood pressure and osteoarthritis. She is a lonely woman who likes to talk. She also has a bad case of "testophilia"—an unnatural affection for medical testing. I suspect that Mrs. Thomasina has never met a doctor she doesn't doubt.

Mrs. Thomasina tests my accessibility day after day. She bypasses my office receptionist when she wants to talk to me. Instead, she phones me at home in the evening. If the line is busy or no one is home, she has the hospital operator page me. Such is the life of a small-town doctor. Her calls never involve an actual emergency; rather, they are about matters that "can't wait." Examples include failing to have a bowel movement the day before, ringing in her ears, a muscle cramp, and unexplained itching.

Mrs. Thomasina has trouble coming to my office. She no longer drives. Her aging children live out of state. She has hired a part-time caregiver to assist her with grocery shopping and household chores. I make home visits every three months to check on Mrs. Thomasina. Her telephone calls bridge the span between house calls and occasional office visits. If a week went by without a call from her, I'd fear she might be dead.

Mrs. Thomasina is apprehensive that there's something terribly wrong with her. In truth, she's much healthier than she imagines. The only way to assuage her concern is to perform some kind of test. Often a urinalysis is enough to satisfy her. I have no inkling what it is about urine that so fascinates Mrs. Thomasina. It is a mystery that ranks up there with Stonehenge and the Bermuda Triangle.

Mrs. Thomasina's lack of confidence in my diagnostic skills is beyond deflating. It's an unintentional insult. As soon as she learns about any medical test (from television or the newspaper or a friend), she must have it. Lately, she's been lobbying me to order a total-body computed tomography (CT) scan for her. I don't know how much longer I can hold out. It's not that I'm worried about the radiation exposure as much as I am about some of the incidental findings that will inevitably cause her additional anxiety and necessitate a further workup.

Money is no object for Mrs. Thomasina when it comes to her health. When the topic of expense is broached, her response is always the same: "I think I'm worth it." She gladly signs all waivers in case Medicare doesn't approve a diagnostic test. She would happily spend her last penny paying for a test. Her faith in technology and medical science approaches religious devotion.

Mrs. Thomasina keeps a notebook of all her medical test results and statistics. It's as thick as an encyclopedia volume. At this week's home visit, she asked me to page through it like a scrapbook. Although she isn't single-handedly bankrupting the health care system, Mrs. Thomasina is definitely putting a small dent in it. I resist as best I can at being her accomplice. God knows I've told Mrs. Thomasina "no" on many occasions when she's asked for tests that I deem medically unnecessary. Yet she has a way of wearing me down. I've suggested cognitive behavioral therapy to her, but she steadfastly refuses. Mrs. Thomasina prefers the life of a test addict.

* * *

Unlike Mrs. Thomasina, Max doesn't worry night and day about staying well. Instead, the 52-year-old laborer has pretty much given up on the likelihood of recovering his good health. Almost a year ago, Max injured his neck at work. He's mad at his employer. He's mad at the workers' compensation insurance company. He's mad at me. I understand his frustration, anger, and distrust. After 11 months of medical treatment, he feels his condition is unimproved. He senses that his boss no longer cares whether he ever returns to work. Max thinks the insurance company is spying on him because it believes he's well enough to resume working.

"Not a bit better," Max announced at his follow-up visit this week. It's the same greeting he has used in the past five office calls.

Without pausing to take a breath, he handed me four pieces of paper and said, "You have to fill these out."

They are insurance forms and temporary disability statements that need to be completed. Max sits on the exam table and seethes. His posture is stiff. He cannot (or will not) move his neck from side to side. He is capable of flexing his neck only about a few centimeters, and even this small change of verticality is accompanied by a grimace and a grunt.

Max is at a point of no return. He has convinced himself that his neck will never improve. He has told me on multiple occasions that he'll never be able to go back to his job. It wasn't that way in the beginning. Back then, he was optimistic and eager to return to work. I still wonder who or what changed his mind—the attorney he hired, the anger he feels at how he's been treated, or his constant pain. Max sees himself as a victim. I used to feel sorry for Max. Now I feel just like him—pessimistic.

Our lack of success is not due to a shortage of effort. Many different kinds of medications have been prescribed and taken. Max is currently on Cymbalta, an antidepressant drug that also reduces the intensity of chronic pain. He doesn't think the medicine is doing him any good, but I see it differently. Whether it is helping his chronic pain or situational depression or both, Max appears a little less irritable even if he isn't any more upbeat about his situation. He also takes pain pills two or three times a day.

It was a struggle getting workers' comp to authorize the Cymbalta. The people there couldn't understand why they should pay for an antidepressant medication. The insurance representative made it clear that the company was only on the hook for treatments related directly to Max's neck injury. I was dumbfounded that they could fail to see the big picture. After lots of phone calls and a little begging on my part, the comp people finally gave in when it became clear I wouldn't give up.

Max has had X-rays and an MRI scan of his neck, nerve conduction studies, an electromyogram (EMG), and even a cervical myelogram. He has seen a neurosurgeon, who advised him that any operation on his neck would be a last resort and not guaranteed to reduce his pain. Max has been through extensive physical therapy and does home cervical traction. He has received steroid injections for his neck. Acknowledging my failure, I referred Max to a pain management program.

"A waste of time," was Max's verdict.

I realize that I'm going to sound like a terrible doctor when I say that I was beginning to think that Max wasn't going to get any better. This week he's finally made me a believer; he's not going to get better. Faith works both ways. A patient has to believe in his doctor and vice versa. Max has given up on me and himself. Neither of us has any expectation now that I will fix his damaged neck. But what about his wounded psyche? Might there still be a chance at healing that?

Now the only thing that brings Max back to see me is the need to complete the workers' compensation forms and receive the pills that briefly and incompletely take away his pain. I remind him that neck problems are unpredictable. There's still a chance that his neck will get better even without surgery. Time might yet do the trick. Still, I am shamed by the lack of conviction in my pep talk. I hardly believe it myself. I recommend that Max keep taking the Cymbalta and continue physical therapy, including a specifically designed work-hardening program to enhance overall fitness and strengthen his muscles. I fill out Max's forms and hand them to him. We nod at one another without speaking a word. What more is there to say? We are both dreading a rerun of today's encounter in three weeks.

*   *   *

A know-it-all, a hypochondriac, and a pain in the neck— Willy, Mrs. Thomasina, and Max—seek only what we all need at one time or another: reassurance, comfort, compassion, and a helping hand. I desperately want to give them all these things and more. Yet despite my efforts, I am unable to deliver the goods. I can't give these patients everything they want. Maybe no one can. I am Don Quixote with an MD degree. I joust with windmills, but my windmills fight back.

How not to care for difficult patients is pretty obvious: don't brush them off. Don't use "stress" as a diagnosis for unexplained symptoms unless you're 99 percent sure that anxiety is an accurate diagnosis and not just a cop-out. Don't be angry. Don't be punitive. Don't propagate despair.

How to care for difficult patients? Inside my office, I know that it involves protocols and limits, truth (including knowing when to admit "I don't know" to yourself and your patient), information and resources, and goals for reasonable results. In my heart, I know time is key. Time is a precious commodity subject to the laws of supply and demand. Difficult patients require more time. Busy doctors find that time is in short supply. Difficult patients are at risk of becoming casualties of the almighty schedule. A 15-minute time slot is hardly enough for complicated patients. No one would make a major decision—choose a spouse, buy a car or a house, select a college, pick a job—after only 15 minutes of deliberation. Why then do we cram important decisions about personal health matters into 15- or 20-minute appointments?

What exactly drives the office schedule of a doctor and dictates how much time is allotted each patient? Multiple considerations, but the big ones include patients' needs, reimbursement, practice volume, hospital responsibilities, a doctor's energy level, and the office staff's desire to get a lunch break and still make it home by 6:00 P.M. When one is dealing with difficult patients, a good case can be made for longer but less frequent office visits.

Extended visits would likely improve patient and physician satisfaction, improve compliance, and upgrade the quality of care. Providing people with more face-to-face time with their doctors does more than merely help communication. Longer visits might actually be more cost-effective than brief ones by reducing the need for frequent follow-up appointments, curtailing the number of consultations and second opinions, decreasing excessive testing, cutting down on the cost of transportation and gas consumption necessitated by repeated short visits with the doctor, and minimizing the amount of missed work for numerous appointments. In this sense, lengthier visits are a bargain. Too bad insurance companies and other payers don't see it that way.

To continue being blunt, it's all about how doctors and patients relate to one another. And the problem with a difficult patient isn't just the patient. It's also the doctor. Difficult patients and their frustrated physicians fail each other. We flop together. We lose hope. And there is no more worthless doctor than one who has lost all hope. Same holds true for a patient.

THE WREATH

Bryan Bordeaux, DO, MPH

Bob (NOT HIS real name) was one my first patients after completing residency. The first time I met him, he reminded me of a scarecrow. He was a thin, unshaven man in his early 70s with clumps of thick brown hair pushing out from underneath his wide-brimmed, straw hat. Adding to the image was a pair of old work suspenders, worn denim jeans, a button-down flannel shirt, and mud-covered rubber boots that went up to his knees. He was the textbook picture of someone with emphysema, having a "pink puffer" appearance complete with the signature pursed lips. Despite this, he was full of life. He was standing in my waiting room beside his wife. Before I could even introduce myself, he interjected in a thick northern New Jersey accent, "Bryan, before you decide to take Jane [also not her real name] and me as new patients, you need to know something. We're complicated."

I thought to myself, "How complicated can they *really* be?" After all, I had just completed my residency and was making final preparations for the boards. As a resident, I was comfortable caring for people with multiple medical problems. At the time, I was building a new practice in rural Pennsylvania and was looking for patients. I was up for the challenge and told them so. They scheduled appointments for another day and were off.

Bob had multiple, chronic medical problems that we "tuned up" over the next six months. We were able to get his breathing a little bit better, his blood pressure and cholesterol lower, and I helped him cut back on his smoking. We developed a great doctor-patient relationship. Frequently, he referred to me as his "quarterback."

Bob was an outwardly affectionate person, demanding a hug after each visit from both my medical students and myself. He often told me that he thought of me as his own son. He and his wife were recent Mennonite converts and became fervent evangelists not only for God, but also for my medical practice. Before long, almost every member of their family and church were also patients of mine.

Early that December, during a routine office visit, he asked me, "So how many wreaths do you want to buy this year?" I had never even known that he sold wreaths. Taken aback, I replied, "Uh, I dunno, hmmm . . . "

Bob cut me off: "Well, my *dentist* buys eight wreaths every year."

"Really?" I responded incredulously, "Why does he need so many wreaths?"

"One for his home and seven to place on the various doors outside his office building."

I felt trapped at this point. "Okay, I'll buy one. How much are they?"

"Forty dollars," Bob stated proudly. That sounded very high to me, and he could read it on my face. "They're really nice wreaths. I pick all of the greens and berries myself. I know just the place in the woods to go. It'll be ready in two weeks."

Two weeks later, Bob delivered the wreath as promised. It was made of lush greens closely packed together with a wide red velvet ribbon and carefully placed bunches of natural red berries and pinecones. It was really one of the nicest wreaths that I had ever seen, and it reminded me of the kind that I would make with my father every winter as a child in rural Massachusetts.

Unfortunately, Bob had a very difficult year ahead of him. I found a large, asymptomatic abdominal aortic aneurysm that required surgical repair. After the procedure, he developed kidney failure and pneumonia. Much to his wife's chagrin, he always wore "that damned hat," even when lying in a hospital bed. His kidneys eventually regained some function, but prolonged bed rest greatly deconditioned him. Despite using continuous oxygen, now he was always short of breath. He also became severely depressed. Despite frequent encouragement, home physical therapy, and antidepressants, his breathing and spirits continued to decline and by late summer, he was largely confined to bed. After a long meeting with him, his family, and his pastor, we all agreed that it was time to begin home hospice.

Paradoxically, after Bob began hospice, his health and mood improved considerably. His life found new meaning as the dying patriarch. Even though he was still largely confined to bed, he established his bedroom as a royal court where he gave decrees and sage advice to all that would enter.

I had made a few house calls for other patients in the past and visited him at home a half dozen times. Bob would call the office frequently with symptoms that needed to be evaluated. Sometimes, when I arrived I found acute medical problems that needed to be addressed, but at other times I found nothing serious and I sensed that he just wanted my companionship.

Early in the fall, as the "quarterback," I developed a game plan to help Bob both physically and emotionally. "Bob," I said casually during a home visit, "I have an idea. I really liked the wreath that you made for me last year. Do you think that you can make another one for me this year?" Suddenly, he smiled and his eyes lit up in a way I had never seen before. "You bet! Bryan, that's a great idea." He slapped his hands together and continued, "But this time, the wreath is free."

Over the next few months, Bob became stronger and stronger by gradually getting out of bed more and by pushing himself to increase his endurance. He never regained most of his stamina, but he was able to take small trips outside the home to go to restaurants with his wife and to come to see me in my office. I kept reminding him about the wreath. Around Thanksgiving, I started to receive progress reports. Everything was coming together right on schedule.

Bob called the office and set up a delivery date. I made sure that my schedule was open to meet with him. Surrounded by his family, he was pushed down the long corridor to my office in a wheelchair with the wreath carefully laid on his lap. Coincidentally, the director of his hospice program, a generous woman named Jennie, paid an unannounced visit to my office at exactly the same time. When she met Bob and his family and heard the story of the wreath, she began to cry. In fact, we all shed a few tears.

The wreath looked similar to the one I had purchased one year before, only it was larger and slightly less manicured. Bob did most of the work himself but admitted receiving a little help from his son-in-law.

After Christmas, Bob again slipped back into depression and became progressively weaker. He fell into a coma and died in late March. I attended his wake, and his family decided to bury him along with his signature hat. Although the wreath was brown at this point and had lost many of its needles, I could not take it down until Bob passed away.

Acknowledgment of
Permissions

"Beyond the White-Coat Ceremony" is reprinted with the permission of Maya Salameh. The story first appeared in the *Yale Journal of Biology and Medicine* 79 (2006).

"Yellow Ooze" is reprinted with the permission of Sarah Canavan. The story first appeared in the *Yale Journal of Biology and Medicine* 80 (2007).

"My Calling" is excerpted from *Routine Miracles*, by Conrad Fischer, and is used with the permission of the author and Kaplan Publishing.

"The Doctor's Wife" is reprinted with the permission of Sayantani DasGupta and the Hastings Center. The story originally appeared in *Hastings Center Report* (March–April 2007).

"Indiscretions" is reprinted with the permission of Anna Reisman and the Hastings Center. The story originally appeared in *Hastings Center Report* (September–October 2005).

READER'S GUIDE

1. Many of the stories deal with the death of a patient. Have you ever experienced death in a professional capacity? If so, how did your approach to it differ from those of the doctors in this book?

2. Do the stories in the collection add a new perspective to your own relationships with physicians, either as a patient or an observer?

3. If you are an internist yourself (or are planning to become one), do the themes and personal stories affect how you see colleagues?

4. In her piece "Human Contact," Rima Bishara explores some of the stark realities of aging. In her interactions

with Mr. and Mrs. T, the author examines the social programs available to people who are elderly and independent, as well as the doctor's responsibility to provide basic human contact. What do you think is the physician's role in a patient's well-being, outside of meeting medical needs?

5. Doug Olson's story "Helping Harry" also takes a look at the physician as a provider of human contact, questioning whether technology can ever replace the doctor-patient relationship. As we see more sophisticated medical technology, what do you see as the balance between medical efficiency and the personal aspects of a face-to-face doctor interaction?

6. In "The Doctor's Wife," Sayantani DasGupta illustrates that a doctor's mind-set extends far beyond the hospital and can affect all aspects of his or her life.

7. In Robert Lamberts's essay, he discusses the sometimes conflicting roles of the doctor as a care provider and the doctor as a businessperson maintaining a thriving practice. When he says "the most important thing I can offer is me," do you agree? Why or why not?

8. Tony Miksanek's essay discusses the challenges of working with "difficult patients" and offers advice for fellow doctors. Do you agree with his tips (*"Don't*

brush them off. Don't use 'stress' as a diagnosis for unexplained symptoms unless you're 99 percent sure that anxiety is an accurate diagnosis and not just a cop-out. Don't be angry. Don't be punitive. Don't propagate despair.")? Are there any you would add to the list, either as a patient or as a fellow health care provider?

9. Conrad Fischer's piece probes the roots of his "calling," treating HIV/AIDS patients and working with legislators and activists to cure the disease and improve patients' quality of life. Have you ever experienced this kind of calling, drawing you toward a vocation? If so, how was it similar to/different from Dr. Fischer's?

10. Tony Miksanek ("On Caring for Difficult Patients") ponders how to approach patients who sometimes don't want to be helped, even though the physician is obligated to treat them. How would you work with someone who doesn't want your help, even when it's in that person's best interests?

About the Editor

MARK TYLER-LLOYD, MD, MPH, received his undergraduate degree in biology from Morehouse College in Atlanta, Georgia. He entered graduate school at New York Medical College in Valhalla, New York, and worked, part-time, as a histologist in the Department of Neuro-pathology, studying multiple sclerosis with a research team. While still in graduate school, he became a counselor on an adolescent unit in a private psychiatric hospital and later the hospital laboratory director. After finishing his graduate degree in Public Health, Dr. Tyler-Lloyd entered Upstate Medical Center in Syracuse, New York, and while there, worked in the Department of Clinical Pathology as a phlebotomist and blood bank technician. Upon finishing his program at Upstate Medical Center, he completed internship and residency in Internal Medicine and Primary Care at the Sound Shore Medical Center of Westchester, a major affiliate of New York Medical College.

While in residency, Dr. Tyler-Lloyd was the first recipient of the Dr. Joseph Lauria Award, given annually to residents who demonstrate the commitment and dedication that Dr. Lauria exemplified during his distinguished career.

Dr. Tyler-Lloyd is currently the director of medical curriculum for Kaplan Medical, and resides in New York.

ABOUT THE CONTRIBUTORS

LEE SAVIO BEERS, MD, is an assistant professor of Pediatrics at Children's National Medical Center and The George Washington University Medical Center. She is the director of the Healthy Generations Program, a "teen-tot" program providing comprehensive medical care, case management, and mental health services to adolescent parents and their children. Dr. Beers received a bachelor of science degree from the College of William and Mary and her medical degree from Emory University School of Medicine. She completed a pediatric residency at Naval Medical Center—Portsmouth. Before coming to Children's Hospital, she worked as a general pediatrician at Naval Hospital—Guantánamo Bay in Cuba and National Naval Medical Center in Bethesda, Maryland. She is a graduate of the George Washington University Graduate School of Education and Human Development Master Teacher Certificate in Medical Education Program.

RIMA BISHARA, MD, is an internist who graduated from medical school in 1986. After finishing residency and chief residency, she served as a doctor in an all-male federal penitentiary for two years. Since then, she has been in solo private practice. In addition to raising two wonderful children with her husband, she volunteers with the American Red Cross, and teaches disadvantaged children and their parents about health and life skills. She created (and continues to develop) the 3Generations Project, a vehicle for getting health information to people who desperately need it. This project was recognized by American Express as a Top 25 Project during the 2008 Members Project contest. In her spare time, she enjoys walking, reading, and writing, ballroom dancing, and riding roller coasters.

BRYAN BORDEAUX, DO, MPH, practices internal medicine in downtown Boston and teaches at Harvard Medical School. After completing his residency in upstate New York, he worked as a National Health Service Corps Scholar in rural Pennsylvania, where he treated patients in a solo office practice, staffed a 22-bed critical access hospital, made house calls, and was featured on a weekly radio program. He went on to complete a general internal medicine fellowship at Johns Hopkins and earned a master of public health degree. In addition to writing, his other interests include health information technology, cooking, baseball, and tennis.

SARAH CANAVAN, MD is a gastroenterologist in Connecticut. She was born in Chicago and completed her undergraduate work at Cornell University, where she studied the interactions of science and society. She received her MD from Cornell University before moving to Yale, where she completed her internship and residency in internal medicine. She continued at Yale as a chief medical resident and then as a fellow in the Section of Digestive Diseases. When not at work, she enjoys running, traveling, and spending time with her family.

SAYANTANI DASGUPTA, MD, MPH, is assistant professor of Clinical Pediatrics and Core Faculty in the Program in Narrative Medicine at Columbia University. She also teaches courses in illness narratives and narrative genetics at Sarah Lawrence College, where she is a prose instructor in their Writing the Medical Experience summer seminar. She is the coauthor of *The Demon Slayers and Other Stories: Bengali Folktales*; the author of a memoir about her education at Johns Hopkins Medical School, *Her Own Medicine: A Woman's Journey from Student to Doctor*; and coeditor of an independently published, award-winning collection of women's illness narratives, *Stories of Illness and Healing: Women Write Their Bodies*. She is an associate editor of the journal *Literature and Medicine*, and her writing has appeared in a variety of publications, including *JAMA*, *Pediatrics*, the *Hastings Center Report*, and the *Journal of Medical Humanities*.

CONRAD FISCHER, MD, is an award-winning medical educator, associate chief of medicine for Educational and Academic Activities at SUNY Downstate School of Medicine, and attending physician at Kings County Hospital in Brooklyn, New York, and a public health advocate. He is the author of numerous USMLE test preparation guides, and he teaches USMLE test preparation for Kaplan Medical.

ROBERT LAMBERTS, MD, works full-time in a private practice in suburban Augusta, GA. He was born in Rochester, NY and attended Houghton College, where he got his BS in chemistry with a minor in music. He then went to Jefferson Medical College in Philadelphia, PA, before completing his residency at Indiana University Hospitals in Indianapolis, IN, where he trained in both internal medicine and pediatrics. He is now board certified in both fields and is a fellow of the American Academy of Pediatrics and a member of the American College of Physicians. Dr. Lamberts is the creator and author of the blog "Musings of a Distractible Mind," a mix of medical observations, discussions on the state of healthcare, personal musings as to what it is really like to be a doctor, and somewhat "quirky" humor.

DAVID A. MATUSKEY, MD, spent his formative years in Orlando, Florida. After graduating from University of South Florida in Tampa with a bachelor's degree in psychology and biology, he joined Peace Corps and was stationed in the oceanic country of Samoa, where he taught biology and physics. On the long way home, he spent time in many Asian countries, which helped formulate his desire to pursue medicine. He enrolled in medical school in Belize the next year, and it was on one of his many clinical rotations that his story is based. After three years of psychiatric residency at the University of Connecticut, he transitioned to Yale University, where he is currently a fellow in clinical neuroscience.

TONY MIKSANEK, MD, is a family physician who has practiced medicine in a small town in Illinois for more than 20 years. In addition, he writes short stories, essays, and book reviews, and he teaches college-level classes on creative writing and modern literature.

DOUGLAS OLSON, MD, grew up in Boston and attended medical school at George Washington University in Washington D.C. He is a resident in Internal Medicine at Yale University. An interest in human rights and social justice is the impetus for his career in the underserved primary care specialty.

ANNA B. REISMAN, MD is a general internist at VA Connecticut, an associate professor at Yale School of Medicine, and co-director of the Yale Internal Medicine Residency Writers' Workshop. She coedited *Telephone Medicine: A Guide for the Practicing Physician* (ACP, 2002). Recent essays and reviews have appeared in *Discover Magazine*,

The New York Times, The Los Angeles Times, Hastings Center Report, and *Lahey Clinic Medical Ethics.*

MAYA SALAMEH, MD, is a graduate of Johns Hopkins University in Baltimore, where she earned a BS degree in Biomedical Engineering. She went on to complete her medical studies at Yale University School of Medicine. After graduation, she chose to stay at Yale for her residency training in internal medicine, where she also served as Chief Resident. "Beyond the White Coat Ceremony" is based on experiences she encountered during her residency. Dr. Salameh is currently Assistant Professor of Clinical Medicine at Columbia University Medical Center, where she specializes in Vascular Medicine. She is the medical director of the Vascular Ultrasound Laboratory and remains actively involved clinical work, research, and the education of medical students and internal medicine residents.

MONIQUE TELLO, MD, MPH, practices primary care women's health at Mass General Hospital in Boston, Massachusetts. She took a meandering route to her current position, via degrees in psychology and comparative literature at Brown, a few years' wandering including much waitressing and a stint teaching STD prevention in Ecuador, medical school at the University of Vermont, a combined med/peds residency at Yale, and a general medicine fellowship with a focus on HIV women's health at Johns Hopkins. She is writing a book about medical training.

ELIEZER VAN ALLEN, MD, is currently an internal medicine resident at the University of California at San Francisco. He was born and raised in Los Angeles, CA, and completed his undergraduate work at Stanford University, where he studied Symbolic Systems. He obtained his medical degree at the University of California—Los Angeles, and he is currently planning on pursuing a career in Hematology/Oncology with a focus on informatics and cancer genetics. During his (rare) free time, he enjoys writing and sleeping, a pastime he has sadly neglected in residency.

HIMALI WEERAHANDI is a fourth-year medical student at Temple University. She plans to pursue a residency in Internal Medicine.

SHARE YOUR STORIES WITH KAPLAN PUBLISHING

K APLAN PUBLISHING, A leading educational resource for doctors, would like to feature your story in an upcoming anthology in the Kaplan Voices: Doctors series. Please share the stories behind the relationships, the experiences, and the issues you've encountered in your medical career—whether you work in a bustling hospital, a rural clinic, private practice, or anywhere in between.

Entertaining and educational, inspirational and practical, each Kaplan Voices: Doctors anthology features true, first-person stories written by doctors themselves, revealing the person behind the white coat.

For writers' guidelines or more information, please contact Kaplan Publishing by email at *kaplanvoicesdoctors@ gmail.com,* or write to us at:

Kaplan Voices: Doctors editor
Kaplan Publishing
1 Liberty Plaza, 24th Floor
New York, NY 10006

Preview

THE REAL LIFE OF A PEDIATRICIAN

Perri Klass, MD

Editor

THE CARE OF STRANGERS

Rachel Kowalsky, MD

A BROTHER AND SISTER have run away from home—or
at least, they wandered away from their grandmother
in the Bronx and took the subway 17 stops, exiting at South
Street Seaport. They were found climbing over a railing to
get a better look at the boats. The brother, Rafael, hands
thrust deep into his pockets, is seven. His sister, Laura,
is four. She wears a raggedy sundress and pink sequined
shoes. Oblivious to the quorum of cops and case workers
their presence has summoned, they were ogling the fish
in the seaport's fish tank.

Their grandmother arrives in the emergency department. She is thin, anxious. She wears thick glasses and
thick heels. I break the news to her—we've had to call
ACS, the Administration for Children's Services, to inves-
tigate the family. Even if the children didn't run away—

even if they only wandered off—they were improperly supervised.

The woman is indignant, frowning at me over her glasses. "We are *buena gente*—good people. You don't know anything about us!"

She's right; I don't know them. In my job as a pediatric emergency physician, I care for thousands of children and families in a year, entering their lives at critical moments and exiting just as quickly. While many patients develop a relationship with their doctor over months and years, a typical ER shift is between 8 and 12 hours—about as long as it takes to fly cross-country, charge a battery, or marinate a chicken. It takes longer for paint to dry on the hospital walls.

The grandmother is interviewed by the ACS social worker. The office door is closed, but I can still hear the escalating emotion from down the hall. Through the shouting and crying, I catch that phrase again: *buena gente*. When she emerges, the grandmother is crying. Laura, the four-year-old,pulls herself away from the fish tank, rushes over, drapes her arms around the old woman's neck, and then starts to cry herself. The woman and child add their tears to the general din of the ER. The medical student I am working with looks at me, distraught. "Maybe we shouldn't have called ACS."

I have a set of rules for taking care of strangers, and I lecture the student about Rule Number One: *Treat every family the same*. In this frenetic setting, I will never learn whether a family is *buena gente* or not, so I have to do the same thing for every little wanderer: call ACS. If the children had strayed from a picnic on the well-heeled Upper East Side, I'd have to do the same (and I have).

Then, because I have a few moments (and the medical student is a captive audience), I share Rule Number Two: *Learn one thing from each patient.* Rafael, the seven-year-old, has a benign heart murmur. I tell her to go and listen to it. That way, when she hears an abnormal murmur, she will know the difference. "See?" I expound. "You'll never see Rafael again, but he will influence your practice for years to come."

Rules one and two are basic. Anyone who went to medical school in the last century has been lectured on both of these topics. The more difficult task, when caring for strangers, is to inject humanity into these brief encounters—to pop in and out of people's lives with grace. Thirty minutes later, when my shift ends, I make an attempt. The children and their grandmother are sitting miserably in an alcove, situated directly between me and the door. "Good-bye," I say, standing uncertainly before them. Nobody looks up. I kneel down to Laura's eye level and offer her a sticker. She scowls at me. I accept my defeat.

The other rule of caring for strangers is one I learned as a resident in pediatrics. It was routine to cross-cover patients, or to care for a patient briefly, usually overnight or on a weekend. On weekdays, each patient had a primary resident, a resident who knew the patient well and was responsible for his or her care. But, despite being called "resident," no doctor truly lives in the hospital—

and when the primary doctor went home, somebody had to assume care of those patients. This is true in essentially every hospital in the country, and it's why the cross-cover role exists. Cross-cover doctors, like ER doctors, must take care of children they do not know.

When I was a resident, we had systems in place to make cross-coverage as seamless as possible. For example, each patient had a weekly log with a column for each day of the week. Each day we recorded the vital signs and lab results, the child's medications and diet specifications, and any important events that had occurred. When we "signed out" a patient to the cross-cover, we handed that doctor the log. It became all-important—the patient's whole illness distilled into a few lines of text.

Despite all the organization, cross-coverage was always a delicate situation. Entering a child's hospital course *in medias res* felt like opening a novel to a random page, or entering a movie theater halfway through the film. I learned to ask a lot of questions at sign-out so that I would never walk into a patient's room unprepared. And I became used to hearing "you don't know my son," or "you don't know what works for my daughter." Experienced parents would even say, as I came by to introduce myself, "I know—you're just cross-covering."

And then, a resident's nightmare: I was cross-covering Amanda Lopez the night she died. Amanda (not her real name) had a rare and virulent form of childhood leukemia. She was DNR (Do Not Resuscitate) and ALOC (Altered Level of Care). The latter meant that we were not to do anything invasive or painful, such as draw blood or put in IVs. She was to receive comfort measures only.

Boyd, my co-resident, signed her out to me. Amanda's primary, Sam, was post-call—he had worked overnight the night before, going home at 11:00 A.M. So Boyd had covered Amanda. And now she was mine: double cross-coverage. She had been febrile all day, lapsing in and out of consciousness, her blood pressure falling. Boyd told me she was going to die. In fact, he had actually started the necessary paperwork for me: the death certificate, the organ donation papers, and the Event Note on the computer—the "event" being death. This is how it read: "Amanda is a 6-year-old female with leukemia. Status: post multiple rounds of chemotherapy, now with end-stage disease and presumed sepsis, on ALOC." I could write the rest later.

Amanda liked to wear ponchos. Her favorite was a nubby cream-colored poncho with navy stripes; it was way too big for her tiny body. I knew her, but not well, the way I knew the kids in my apartment building. She had been in the hospital a long time. Her log had weeks and weeks worth of papers stapled together, but since she'd become ALOC, not much was written there. She had hollow cheeks, large, lovely eyes, and a wise, pointed chin. She was very close with her oncologist and with Sam, her primary—but neither of them was there. I was there.

I introduced myself to Amanda's parents. I said I was their doctor for the night. I asked whether Amanda was comfortable and if they needed anything. Amanda's mom asked whether Sam, her primary resident, was around. I said no. He was actually at a wedding, but I couldn't bring myself to say this. She nodded. I suppose on the scale of disappointments, this final one was small. She asked me for a glass of water for Amanda. *Ice?* I asked. *No thanks.* I stood around for a bit, watching her offer the water to Amanda. I remember that the girl's lips were dry, that she didn't drink anything, and that her mom carefully applied some lip balm. Amanda lay on her side, propped up on pillows, a nasal cannula delivering oxygen with a soft whir. Her parents lay in bed too—one on either side of her. Nobody spoke to me or looked at me, so I left the room.

If Amanda's life was a novel, I was a minor character—a character without lines. I sat at the nurse's station, wondering what I could do for her. My pager went off all night, calling me to other rooms and other patients, but I kept returning to the desk outside Amanda's room. "Do you think they need me?"

Amanda's nurse shook her head. "Best to leave them alone."

It was torture not to go in the room. Shouldn't I know the patient whose final Event Note I was to write? Shouldn't there be a moment of connection? Well, I had brought her a cup of water. Somehow that made me feel better.

I checked on Amanda twice more. The first time, she was cuddling with her mother. The second time, she appeared to be asleep. An hour or two later, her nurse called me. "I think she passed," she said. She was crying. Another nurse hugged her. I stood awkwardly, my hands in the pockets of my white coat. "Go on in," she said. "You have to pronounce her."

So that was my job—to listen to Amanda's quiet chest and confirm that she was gone. I put my stethoscope over her heart and listened for a long time. When I looked up, both parents were watching me. It was a strange moment, the three of us in the room with Amanda. I opened my mouth to speak, but they cut me off. They reached for each other. And that was the end of the story.

From Amanda, I learned Rule Number Three: *family first*. I don't think her parents remember me. They probably remember Sam, and their favorite nurse. I was just the one with the stethoscope, at the end—an extra in Amanda's story, and the story of her family.

But in my own story, Amanda is a prominent figure. Because of her, I learned Rule Number Four: *12 hours is just the beginning*. Because I still think about Amanda Lopez, and it's five years later.

Don't give up. The last rule, Rule Number Five. It's weeks later, and I am back in the ER with another medical student, telling him what I like about my job. The level of acuity, the interesting cases, the varied age groups. The many dramas, big and small, that come through my door each day. The medical student plans to go into General Pediatrics because, he says, he likes the continuity of care. He wants to get to know his patients.

I defend my profession. Children with respiratory ill-ness often come back for a "resp check"—a second visit—and babies with fevers commonly are brought back to the ER for a follow-up visit as well. If we put in stitches, we usually take them out. I enjoy these reunions, the familiar faces, the "how are you doing?"

And even though there are many patients we never see again, I tell the student, *don't give up.* After all, a lot can be accomplished in just a few hours. Parties start and end. Entire weather systems change. Shakespeare's plays are just hours long, and think of all that happens there—people fall in love, wage war, return from exile. Kingdoms fall.

And, can you believe it? That same day, I bump into the grandmother at the end of my shift. We are both in the lobby, trying to exit the hospital through the revolving door. There are several people ahead of us, and we wait awkwardly together.

Finally, she nods at me.

"The kids?" I ask, looking around. She tells me she is here alone, visiting a sick relative.

"How are they?"

"*Malcriados.*" Poorly behaved.

"I'm sorry..." I begin.

She enters the revolving door, waving away my apol-ogy. "The woman came from ACS, she checked the house, she talked to us—and she left. She saw we were good people."

"I try to treat every family the same," I say, defending myself as I stumble through the door behind her.

She stands and faces me in the bright sunlight. Then, she surprises me. "You did the right thing," she says. "If somebody had done that for my brother and me when we were young, it might have saved his life." And just like that, she strides off in her thick heels. The whole conversation is two minutes from start to finish—about as long as it takes to adjust to the winter light, shake my head, and watch her disappear down the broad avenue.

Forsan

Dipesh Navsaria, MD, MPH, MSLIS

Forsan et haec olim meminisse juvabit.
(Perhaps someday you will rejoice to recall even this.)
— Virgil, *The Aeneid*, Book I

I T WAS 8:00 on a December morning, just a couple of
days before Christmas. My last pre-vacation call night
in the newborn intensive care unit was drawing to a
close. This particular night had been worrisome. I had
two very small preemies side-by-side in one corner of the
unit, both, oddly enough, with the same first name. One,
J.R., had been my patient since I had come on service,
and was still very tenuous and struggling to gain weight
in the face of not only her prematurity, but also a patent

ductus arteriosus (PDA), an opening between the pulmonary artery and the aortic arch, a remnant of fetal circu-
lation that refused to close despite medication.

J.D., the other baby, had a similar story, and occupied
the bed spot next to J.R. She wasn't one of "ours," but was
a transfer from another hospital, who had come to us with
the same open ductus, also persisting in the face of several
rounds of medication. The plan had been for them both
to have their PDAs ligated, or tied off surgically on the
same day, while the surgeon, staff, and equipment were
all available. This had happened the previous morning,
and both had done well through their early postoperative
course.

I checked on them both multiple times through the
night, and was reassured—mostly. J.R. was doing okay, but
J.D. had some oddly low blood pressures at times, though
then they would come back up on their own. The nurse
and I agonized over her on an hourly basis and promised
each other to keep a close watch. The neonatologist had
stayed in-house that night, and he had come by to check
on both babies several times as well. We looked them over,
discussed the numbers, and opted to continue to watch,
albeit a bit nervously. I was glad he was there, because it
wasn't a clear-cut situation—in cases such as this, years of
experience and judgment are important.

As the dawn approached, a sense of relief spread over
me. The long night was over, and after post-call morning
rounds, I would be able to go home and enjoy a well-
deserved few days off in the midst of my busy intern year.

I started going from patient to patient, getting my numbers together, double-checking my calculations in the post-call haze. I was checking labs on the computer in the resident work area when, suddenly, everything went bad.

The neonatology fellow came striding out and declared that J.D. was "one sick little kid." He showed me the printout from the routine morning blood gas that had just been drawn. While I'm sure there have been lower pH values in the NICU before, this was the lowest I'd ever seen. There are many reasons for a low pH, but in essence, the blood becoming this acidic is a sign that something is profoundly wrong—this was the cry of millions of stressed cells struggling against some great duress. What was particularly remarkable was that there was no change in her vitals or clinical exam at this point.

What followed felt like a massive blur—in some ways, it lasted only a few minutes; in others, it was endless. It was not long before J.D.'s clinical status started to deteriorate. She went into cardiac arrest. The neonatologist who had come on service that morning called a code, and around the baby's tiny, less-than-three-pound body we had about nine people. By some stroke of luck, we had the NICU pharmacist on hand, and a pediatric cardiologist who was doing an echocardiogram on another patient rolled the machine over and gave us an intra-code look at her cardiac function.

Despite the blur, I remember the looks on people's faces. I saw J.R.'s parents, huddled by their own baby's incubator, trying their best not to look at us but fully, acutely, and terribly aware that there was a life-and-death drama going on—with a child who just had the same procedure as their little girl.

I was grateful that J.D.'s parents had come in, just before she began to deteriorate. I told them about the blood gas then, but I don't think they entirely processed how serious this was. I recall them standing back as we started chest compressions. I myself could barely tell what was going on with the code as the neonatologist called out orders, but I did my best to keep them updated as they watched us start the compressions.

There was a giddy moment when we brought back the baby's heart and restored a normal rhythm. A small cheer went up, although there was always the unspoken question: how long had her little brain been without sufficient oxygen? Granted, neonates are incredible and their physiology can bounce back from situations that would have long ago killed you or me, but there are limits.

This, however, was not to be. Within a few minutes, she decompensated again, and we were back to manually ventilating her lungs and compressing her chest. We had been working on her for almost three hours when I saw the attending's face contort and her voice crack as she raised the possibility that it was time to stop. I knew this point had been coming for a long time, but I hadn't quite believed it until now, and I felt a lump form in my throat. The attending went over to talk to the parents and reviewed the situation, then raised that final, awful question that no parent should ever have to hear.

Their answer was that we should stop. I knew—we all knew—that this was the right thing at this point. I've never been one to endorse fighting on in the face of over-whelming odds. But for a patient that was doing reasonably well...how awful! I thought about how they had brought their child to our hospital after getting her through those tenuous early weeks, and how they would be leaving with-out her. I can't possibly imagine exactly how they felt, but I'd like to believe that I tried my best to attend to their needs during the code, and I had spent much of the night watching over their daughter.

We cleared away the excess lines and medical equip-ment and prepared to move the baby so we could let the parents hold her as she slipped away. Once she was clear of her attachments to the medical world, I started to lift her, ready to turn and give her to her grieving parents. I found myself being stopped by one of the senior nurses, who had J.D.'s nurse step in and lift her, saying to me, "She's his nurse."

The mixed feelings of sadness, anger, and bewilder-ment washed over me. Yes, that was true, but why did that matter? I had been there at that point for 29½ long hours, and I felt I had some clear right to participate in the last moments of this child. Perhaps I was being selfish, or petty, but the message I got was that because I was a physician, I didn't have the authority to care.

This might not surprise those who are used to medical environments where there is an antagonistic relationship between nursing and medical staff. However, it did me—I generally got along with the NICU nurses very well, and there was seldom cause for disagreement or bickering. I didn't expect to be booted out of this process quite like this. My own hope to join in the parents' grieving for just a moment was kicked to the curb.

I stepped back, yielding to a group of four nurses who surrounded J.D.'s mother, arranging blankets and pillows. Helpless and with no one around me, I turned to the wall and began sobbing into my arm. After a few moments, I exited the NICU to the privacy of the resident call room and wept.

I was not as alone as I might have thought—bless their hearts, my two senior resident colleagues who had come in that morning and assisted with the code saw me leaving in tears and came to check on me. One of them, upon realizing that these were the last hours before I started vacation, took my notes from me and told me to go home. After 30 hours and the emotional exhaustion of watching a patient I'd agonized over die, I did so, following some brief, feeble words of protest, of course.

To this day, I'm grateful for their clear-headed words and compassion. Why? Because, as deeply as this death affected me, no one else ever said anything that acknowledged my pain or the stake that I had in this patient.

While I'd had patients die before, as a student, my connection to them didn't happen to be particularly close. One patient of mine died when I was a physician assistant—but well, it all happened in another hospital, away from me, and I wasn't even involved in treating the illness that led to her demise. Residency, however, brings a great and terrible intensity to everything. The sheer crush of time spent in any one particular setting magnifies both the joy and despair of caring for patients.

A week later, when I returned to work, I was chatting with a couple of the nurses when one of them referred to J.D.'s death and began to tell me about it. The other nurse broke in, reminding her that I had been there, not just in the morning, but through the whole night. Was I that invisible?

A few months later, while discussing another case with the attending who had been there in the morning, I had to remind her that I had been there for the entire thing. Was I so interchangeable that my presence there as a person meant nothing?

Medical education has slowly evolved over time, and the old-time dichotomy between medicine and nursing has blurred in both directions. And while the task of being a resident often means having lesser "stakes" in a patient than when you're an attending, there is certainly emotional investment in our patients. I'd like to believe that I'm a caring, involved physician. I'd like to hope that I do the right things. But to be locked out by old assumptions and lines in the sand—well, a small part of me died with that little girl that morning.

Some redemption did come, in a sense, almost two years later. As the resident covering the regular nursery, I had just come on duty for the overnight shift. I walked into another drama, again of the type that only the NICU can generate. A child who had been born two days earlier had suffered a period of hypoxia and was clearly brain-dead, as verified by an EEG. The family, after long deliberation, had made the choice to withdraw life-sustaining care, although they were waiting for one more family member, who had been delayed by bad weather, to arrive from out of town. The baby, M, forced the issue by dislodging her endotracheal tube. The attending asked the family whether they wanted us to reintubate or to withdraw care at this point.

Once again, I remember their faces. The baby's mother contorted in tears, sobbing, saying that she couldn't go through this again. The baby's father, taciturn but also in pain, made the final statement that we should withdraw care. Again, just as two years prior, we began to remove lines and prepare to give a child to her parents for her final time with them.

I had just walked in on this situation, and I had little to no emotional connection with this patient. The other resident (who was actually assigned to the NICU) was a cross-cover and didn't know this family either. So, to some extent, I readied myself for being pushed out of the situation. I even stepped back to let the baby's nurse give her to her parents. They were allowed to take her to the family room, where they could sit, hold her, and spend their last moments together. I wandered away, my presence clearly unneeded at this point.

It was, however, not 15 minutes later that her nurse came and found me.

"The family thinks she's gone."

I quickly looked around, but the neonatologist and the NICU resident were nowhere nearby, probably attending to other pressing matters. I didn't want to do something that was technically the job of the NICU resident, but at the same time, I didn't want to leave this family waiting in the great pause between the moments that their child was living and dead.

I took a deep breath and asked the nurse to grab a neonatal stethoscope, and we walked to the room together. I rehearsed in my head precisely what I needed to do and say—this family would always remember this moment, and the words that came out of my mouth. We walked in and I briefly said hello, with nods and looks of concern; my reason for being there required no announcement. I uncovered the baby's small, untimely stilled chest and listened for a while, the silence filling my ears. I looked at the clock and simply, quietly, pronounced her dead, for the first time in my career.

The parents exhaled as if they'd been holding their breath, and relief filled their faces. I sat with them for a moment, holding their hands and offering my condolences. The room was not filled with grief and agony as it had been at the moment they decided to withdraw care, but rather with a small, quiet sense of stillness and release. We walked out, and later her nurse found me and thanked me for how I had handled things.

I don't know why this was different. Certainly there were obvious contrasts; M's parents' had expected her to die, while J.D. had taken a sudden, unexpected turn for the worse. A planned, compassionate withdrawal of support is a very different ending from a code situation, with its feelings of failure and defeat. And, of course, the personalities of the people involved change and mesh in different ways. Or maybe there was some difference in me over those two years, some evolution. I don't know for sure.

Not for a second do I believe that these losses are truly mine; the tragedies belong to the grieving families, but there is undoubtedly a connection left asunder between provider and patient. The cold, objective perspective we learn in medical school doesn't always hold true—we contain human feelings: ego, love, compassion, and grief. In the act of bearing witness to others' loss, I can salute and honor that which once was and that which now is.

I do know, however, that after every death I hear about, I go out of my way to find my fellow residents and interns (as well as medical students), make sure they're okay, and let them know that if they need to talk, I'm here.

Baptism by Fire

Alenka Zeman, MD

I FELT THAT THERE was something different about that
bleak day even before it started. I woke up before the
sun had a chance to rise, and drove in the cold winter
morning to the community hospital where I was spending
a month as the supervising resident. A trip that normally
took close to an hour on those slippery winter mornings
took me only 30 minutes this time. For some reason, there
were no traffic jams, breakdowns, or ice between me and
the hospital. In hindsight, it feels as though fate was beckoning me to the hospital.

As an overworked resident, my first emotion when
I stepped into the hospital that morning was frustration. "I could still be in bed," I muttered to myself as
the glass front doors to the hospital creaked open. The
cafeteria was not even open yet, so I couldn't grab a cup

of coffee. Lacking sufficient caffeine, I shuffled upstairs and plopped myself in front of a computer, hoping that I would be invisible for 30 minutes until I could get a sign-out report on the patients from the overnight doctor.

I hoped I would have a brief respite, but a little later, I heard my intern (a first-year resident) storm into the room. "Wow," I thought. "She's here early too." Her voice was hesitant as she struggled to get my attention. "There was a kid admitted last night with gastroenteritis." I barely looked up from my computer.

Gastroenteritis is a viral illness that causes vomiting and diarrhea. It swarms the pediatric floors during the winter, and is one of the most common illnesses we take care of as residents. In fact, we consider it a rite of passage to come down with profuse diarrhea before we graduate. So, of course it wasn't out of the ordinary to see an admission with that diagnosis at this time of year. "Do you think you could come take a look at him?" she asked. "He has this funny breathing pattern, as if he has diabetes." The intern's voice grew more urgent, but what she was saying was inconsistent with the normal blood sugar level I had seen on the computer lab list for this patient. I looked up from the computer and was about to explain to her that there was no way this child had diabetes, when I saw the worried look on her face. I knew then that I had to go and see the child for myself.

I will never forget the feeling in my chest when I walked into that child's room with my intern trailing behind me. It was dark, but in the distant corner I could see a large metal crib with tall hospital rails on the side. Inside the crib was a very thin two-year-old child, with floppy blond hair, lying rigid and flat on his back. His arms were straight at his side and he kept extending them in an odd, repetitive motion. This was something I had been taught to recognize in medical school but had never seen in real life. It was a situation that I had hoped I would never see, because it meant that he was posturing from swelling in his brain. As I entered the room I had expected to see a mother or father at the bedside. Instead, I saw an older man and woman, likely the grandparents, sitting in the corner with a four-year-old sibling draped on their knees. The grandmother whispered, "Please don't disturb him. He is finally sleeping peacefully."

My heart sank again, because I realized I didn't even know this child's first name. I had never met these people before, and now somehow, in a matter of seconds, I had to express to them that their grandchild was very sick, that he could die, and that they needed to trust me. But why should they trust me? I didn't know much, if anything, about their grandchild outside of the dire situation that he was in. I was only in my second year of pediatric residency, but one of the big lessons we learn early on is to recognize sick children versus not-sick children. At the time, I wasn't sure how I was going to help this child, but I knew I had to do something fast—or he was going to die.

I ran to the side of the crib and used all my strength to lower those creaky iron rails that flanked it. I picked up the child, and his weak, exhausted body just sank into my arms. I left my intern to explain to the grandparents what was happening and rushed with the child to the treatment room, where I could gather nurses and equipment. I was unable to make eye contact with the family as I left the room. Maybe I didn't want to see their scared faces, or perhaps I did not want them to see how petrified I was.

Acute cerebral herniation, or brain swelling, is something that we all learn how to manage in medical school—but it is rarely something that you deal with in real life unless you have chosen to become a brain surgeon. It is definitely rarely encountered in a small community hospital like the one where I, as a second-year resident, was the doctor in charge. When I chose pediatrics as a career, I was hoping that I would never have to deal with acute neurological emergencies like this, but there was no avoiding it now.

The next 15 minutes felt like an out-of-body experience. I stood at the head of the bed calling out orders, but my mind kept fixating on the fact that a child's life was in my hands. I could hear myself calling a "Code Blue," which signified that this child was dangerously close to death and that I needed help. The room began to fill with nurses and other doctors who were ready to help out. Everyone started falling into his or her role: the anesthesiologists were putting a tube down the patient's throat to help him breathe; one nurse was drawing blood and starting more lines in the patient; another nurse was pushing the medications to try to stop his brain from swelling; and a handful of other assistants were hustling in and out of the room, bringing more supplies. Even the medical students were standing at attention in the corner, ready to help out if something was needed. I seemed to be calling out orders one by one, but I couldn't even follow what I was saying, as my heart and brain both seemed to be racing at warp speed.

My intern thrust a cell phone to my ear, and fortunately, there was a very calming voice on the other end. "I know you can do this. We have talked about what to do in this situation," the voice said. It was the pediatric intensive care unit fellow in my own hospital, the major hospital about 45 minutes away in the center of the city. "Just get him stabilized. I am mobilizing the flight team to come pick him up." Of course, I knew that if I were sitting in the middle of a lecture at the hospital, calmly sipping a cup of coffee, I would be able to quickly recount the steps a resident would need to go through in this situation. None of my training had prepared me for how I would feel when I saw a young child unresponsive because of the acute changes in his brain.

Out of the corner of my eye, I saw a figure dressed in black approach the doorway. I turned and saw the child's grandfather, with tears cascading over the wrinkles in his face. He was leaning on the shoulder of a priest as they tiptoed into the room together. "My grandchild has never been baptized. I need for him to be baptized...just in case." There was no question that the grandfather understood the seriousness of this moment. I silently nodded, and the sea of nursing staff parted for the priest and grandfather to slip to the head of the bed. Drops of water splattered on the child's fore-head, and a sense of tranquility filled the room as everyone stopped for a few seconds to watch the ceremony. The priest uttered the child's name for the first time: "Timothy."

The moment of silence was interrupted by a booming voice announcing that the CT scanner was ready. We needed to wheel the child downstairs for imaging, so that we could better understand why his brain had swelled so suddenly. I gently peeled the grandfather's fingers off his grandchild. "We need to go now, but I promise he will be in good hands," I whispered softly. The grandfather and I made eye contact for the first time.He did not speak, but with his silent nod I knew he was trusting me to take care of his grandchild.

When the image appeared on the monitor next to the CT scanner, there was no need for the radiologist to explain to the crowd what we saw. There was a huge mass in the posterior aspect of the brain. A brain tumor. The story started to fall into place. My intern had by then contacted the child's parents, who were away on vacation, and they had reported that he would throw up every morning. This caused him to lose a significant amount of weight. The grandparents had come to visit and noticed these symptoms, and thus wisely brought him to the hospital to be evaluated. Every pediatrician fears that a case of vomiting will be dismissed as a mere virus, when in reality the child has an undiagnosed brain tumor. In fact, this is a very rare turn of events, but Timothy's case was one of those exceptions.

The door opened and four people in bright blue flight suits with red backpacks appeared. In a morning that had already been filled with religious moments, I couldn't help thinking that angels had arrived. The med flight team was here. They quickly and efficiently assumed the care of the child, loaded him on the stretcher, and whisked him off to the helicopter. I knew that in about ten minutes, Timothy would be landing on the roof of the intensive care unit, where a crew of neurosurgeons would be waiting eagerly to assume his care.

After the child was safely en route to the bigger hospital, the doctors and nurses in the treatment room were gone just as quickly as they had arrived. Before I knew it, I was standing by an empty stretcher in a room littered with supplies, with nothing but my thoughts to keep me company. What if the grandparents had not brought him in to the hospital the night before? He probably would have died at home in his sleep. What if the traffic patterns had changed and my intern had not been here to check on him early in the morning? And now, what will his overall prognosis be?

I leaned my head on the stretcher, and the tears that I had been holding back all morning came flowing out. I wasn't sure whether they were tears of sadness, relief, or even joy because I could actually say that I had saved the life of a child. All I knew was that it felt good to release some of my pent-up emotions. As I wiped off my face, I knew that I had to get back to caring for the other 15 children on the floor. And the team would be waiting for me to discuss what had happened. I exited the room, but before I left, I looked back to the spot where I had seen a child baptized and realized that I, too, had been baptized, by fire.